THE HOLISTIC FIBROMYALGIA TREATMENT PLAN

THE HOLISTIC
FIBROMYALGIA
TREATMENT PLAN

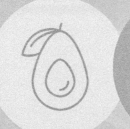
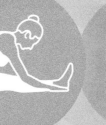

28-Day Plans for Healthy Digestion, Therapeutic Movement, and Emotional Well-Being

Dr. Amarilis Méndez

ROCKRIDGE
PRESS

Interior and Cover Designer: Gabe Nansen
Art Producer: Janice Ackerman
Editors: Clara Song Lee, Andrea Leptinsky
Production Editor: Ashley Polikoff
Custom Illustration: © 2020 Remie Geoffroi: pp: 47, 124-143; © 2019 Charlie Layton: p. 42, 43, 53. Cover Illustration: left icon: Kilroy79/istock
Author photo courtesy of © Revolver Photography
ISBN: Print 978-1-64739-503-2

eBook 978-1-64739-328-1

R0

To everyone who feels, or has felt, hopeless due to a chronic mental or physical condition, never lose hope and never give up. Your breakthrough may be just beyond your point of greatest despair.

CONTENTS

INTRODUCTION

I was a college student when it started to feel like everything was falling apart. I had suffered from insomnia and migraines since I was thirteen, and I had learned to grit my teeth and get through various forms of chronic pain. Now in my early twenties, I was studying biology and working two jobs to support myself, and everything about my life was overwhelming. I developed chronic anxiety. By my sophomore year, my pain had become so widespread that at times I could barely function. I finally sought medical help and immediately hit an obstacle: doctors couldn't explain what was wrong with me.

I kept returning to doctors and going to the emergency room and getting the same non-answers. Doctors ran tests on me that came back "normal," and they started to question my sanity. Even I did. Medical professionals told me I couldn't have those symptoms I was describing. They would ask me if maybe it was just stress or if I needed to see a psychiatrist.

Doctors gave me narcotics to ease the pain, and at night I needed sleep meds but nothing really made me feel normal. They couldn't tell me why I had so much pain, but they were willing to keep writing prescriptions—I felt like I was being experimented on, and I wanted nothing to do with it anymore.

After almost seven frustrating years, I finally got a diagnosis: I had fibro-myalgia. I'd been dismissed as a crazy person and a hypochondriac, and it was cathartic to have someone acknowledge at last that the pain wasn't all in my head and that something real was wrong with me. Still, the answer didn't give me much hope. I believed fibromyalgia was a condition with no cure. I learned that the known treatments might not work, and I saw a list of drugs with horrible side effects. There was a possibility that I wouldn't be able to work and support myself. One doctor told me I probably wouldn't get better and that I might have to apply for disability. Sometimes I would go through my days feeling like a zombie.

But I was determined to find another way to live the rest of my life. Although my original plan was to become a medical examiner, I decided to study natural medicine in hopes that I could learn something that would help me. Over several years, I was able to use what I learned to heal my own body. And working as a naturopath, I have helped others overcome or prevent chronic illness.

I have developed this guide for readers who are ready to be proactive about their healing process but don't know where to begin.

In this book you will find:

- Practical four-week plans to help you improve rest, emotional health, digestion, and physical movement.
- Easy recipes that require few ingredients and minimal preparation time.
- Natural remedies for common symptoms experienced by people with fibromyalgia.
- Ways to manage a health-conscious lifestyle with limited income and resources.

CHAPTER 1
UNDERSTANDING FIBROMYALGIA

After being diagnosed with this condition, the first step is to gain an understanding of what the condition is, what causes it, and what can be done to find relief. Sometimes the medical jargon can be overwhelming and difficult to understand. Fortunately, with a thorough understanding of the basics, you will be equipped to begin your journey to relief. This chapter will go over what is currently known about fibromyalgia.

BIG-PICTURE BASICS

People with fibromyalgia experience widespread musculoskeletal pain, fatigue, sleep disturbances, and problems with their memory and moods; they might experience symptoms like "fibro fog," which makes it hard to focus. Fibromyalgia is a common, chronic widespread pain disorder, and according to an analysis of the 2012 National Health Interview Survey, nearly four million people in the United States have the condition. Researchers now believe that it may stem from a disruption in the brain's ability to process pain, which makes the body much more sensitive not only to pain but also to other sensory experiences like touch, temperature, and sound. In a scientific article published in *Mayo Clinic Proceedings*, several members of the Fibro-Collaborative—a group of experts on the condition—wrote that it was as if fibromyalgia turned up the volume on pain signals.

Women are much more likely to have this condition than men, and the average age range at the time of diagnosis is 35 to 45. However, many people say they've had symptoms, including chronic pain, that started long before they received their diagnosis. The condition may develop suddenly after a stressful or traumatic event or injury, or the symptoms may appear gradually and become more severe as time goes by.

Stuck in a Stress Response

With fibromyalgia, the body is stuck in a stress response. In response to stress, your body releases cortisol, a steroid hormone that plays a vital role in many bodily functions such as metabolism, blood pressure, memory formation, and anti-inflammatory responses. Cortisol levels normally fluctuate throughout the day, with the highest levels in the morning and a steady decrease until nighttime. In times of chronic stress, the body has elevated levels of cortisol for an extended period of time. Chronic stress depletes the immune system, anti-pain system, and antianxiety system. It can impair cognitive function, decrease bone density and muscle tissue, and increase abdominal fat. These are all issues commonly experienced with fibromyalgia.

UNDERLYING ISSUES OR TRIGGERS

Although the precise causes of fibromyalgia are unknown, there is evidence that genetic factors may contribute to developing this condition and that it may be triggered by certain infections. Some studies have found that fibromyalgia is more common in people with the conditions listed below. Because there is evidence of a possible genetic component to fibromyalgia, it's possible that these infections or traumas activate genes. More research needs to be done to confirm these potential underlying issues.

Hepatitis C: A viral infection, hepatitis C is spread through infected blood. It causes liver inflammation and can sometimes lead to serious liver damage. This infection is now treatable, but it's possible for many people to be asymptomatic. Recent research indicates there could be a link between hepatitis C infection and fibromyalgia.

Adrenal insufficiency: Adrenal insufficiency occurs when the adrenal glands do not produce enough cortisol and can cause fatigue, difficulty regulating blood sugar and blood pressure, and increased pain and anxiety.

Candida overgrowth: Candida is a fungus naturally found in the intestines that, in excess, can cause pain, brain fog, skin issues, fatigue, digestive issues, pain, mood swings, and recurrent fungal infections.

Food intolerances/sensitivities: These are non-allergic responses to foods that can cause or increase pain, skin issues, digestive issues, and fatigue, among other symptoms.

Genetic mutations: Mutations, or alterations, to the MTHFR gene can inhibit your body's natural detoxification pathways. Increased toxicity in the body can cause pain, brain fog, fatigue, poor immunity, and general malaise.

Heavy metal toxicity: Heavy metal toxicity can occur after exposure to environmental pollutants, amalgam dental fillings, and consuming fish with high mercury levels, and can cause chronic fatigue, digestive issues, brain fog, and chronic aches and pains.

Leaky gut: Leaky gut occurs when the small gaps in the intestinal wall become loose, allowing for increased permeability. Symptoms of leaky gut include digestive issues, skin issues, fatigue, and food sensitivities.

Mycotoxins: These are toxins produced by molds, and when they are in our bodies, they can cause several neurological symptoms like numbness, tingling, twitching, chronic pain, sleep disturbances, lowered immunity, and general malaise.

Thyroid hormone imbalance: Less than optimal levels of thyroid hormones can cause fatigue, depression, constipation, brain fog, and sleep disturbances.

Nutrient deficiencies: Deficiencies in several different nutrients can cause increased pain, fatigue, muscle stiffness, general malaise, sleep disturbances, anxiety, and many other symptoms.

COMMON COEXISTING CONDITIONS

There are several conditions that are common in people with fibromyalgia; many of them have symptoms that overlap with fibromyalgia. It is important to discuss these with your healthcare provider, since it will influence your treatment options.

Anxiety and depression: Many people with fibromyalgia experience anxiety, depression, or both, which can make it harder to find the motivation to do anything or cope with their illness.

Chronic fatigue syndrome: With this condition, which is also called myalgic encephalomyelitis, a person experiences extreme, long-term fatigue that interferes with their everyday life. They may have other symptoms, including memory problems, headaches, and sensitivity to noise.

Headaches/migraines: These are headaches that can be accompanied by nausea, weakness, and sensitivity to light, sound, and smell. People may see an "aura"—some kind of visual disturbance that signals the onset of a migraine.

Irritable bowel syndrome: This disorder is characterized by constipation and/or diarrhea, abdominal bloating, cramping, pain, and gas.

Lupus: This autoimmune disorder can be mild or severe. The body's immune system attacks its own tissues. Common symptoms include joint and muscle pain, red rashes, fever with no known cause, and hair loss.

Insomnia: Insomnia is a sleep disorder in which a person has trouble falling asleep or staying asleep for several nights each week. Lack of sleep will exacerbate other issues, so addressing this will enhance your ability to heal.

Restless leg syndrome (RLS): RLS causes an uncontrollable urge to move the legs, often to relieve a feeling of discomfort. People usually experience the symptoms of RLS while sitting or lying down in the evening or at night, making it hard to sleep.

Rheumatoid arthritis: Unlike osteoarthritis, which is associated with aging, rheumatoid arthritis is an autoimmune disease in which the immune system attacks the body's tissues, leading to swelling and pain.

Sleep apnea: People with sleep apnea often snore loudly, and the condition leads people to repeatedly stop breathing during sleep. This disrupts the ability to rest. Sleep apnea is a potentially serious condition that can lead to heart problems and, in rare cases, death.

Temporomandibular joint disorder (TMJ): The temporomandibular joint connects the jawbone to the skull; people with TMJ have pain or tenderness in the jaw.

PARTNERING WITH HEALTHCARE PROVIDERS

Achieving optimal health is a team effort. Your healthcare provider is the expert in diagnostics and treatment options, but their ability to help you will also depend on how well you are able to communicate your health concerns and goals. No one knows your body as well as you do. Talking to your doctor about your symptoms and needs will equip them to give you the best recommendations. Ideally, you want a healthcare provider who encourages open communication, educates you as much as possible, and honors your beliefs and desires. Here are a few tips on creating this type of collaborative relationship:

1. **Find the right healthcare provider for you.** When choosing your healthcare provider, remember the three Cs: competent (you trust your doctor to be an expert in their field); compassionate (you feel your doctor truly cares about you and wants you to get well); and collaborative (your doctor sees you as their partner in figuring out what will work best for you).

2. **Keep a personal medical record/journal.** Having a written record of everything will ensure that you give thorough and accurate information to your healthcare provider. Writing down your experiences is a good idea for people dealing with any illness, but it's especially important for people with fibromyalgia because the condition can lead to memory problems. This book will provide charts and worksheets to assist with journaling.

3. **Be honest with your provider.** Consult with your provider before starting or stopping any course of treatment, including the recommendations in this book. Also, give your provider feedback on their recommendations. Let them know when you feel something was helpful, neutral, or detrimental. Be as sincere and detailed as possible to ensure they have a better understanding of your concerns and goals.

Survival Guide: "My Healthcare Provider Isn't Helpful"

Sometimes you may find yourself dissatisfied with your healthcare provider. Perhaps you feel your provider is unsupportive or dismissive. You deserve a practitioner you trust; you deserve to see them regularly and to build a relationship. You can contact the National Fibromyalgia Association for resources that will help you find a "fibro-friendly" doctor. Additionally, you should look for fibromyalgia or chronic pain support groups in your area (see page 146 for recommended resources). People in these groups have had many of the same experiences you've had, and they may have recommendations for local healthcare providers. Realistically, you and your doctor may not always agree on what is best for you. Always ask questions, do your own research on reputable health websites, and share the information with your provider. If you feel like you are not being heard, or if you don't feel comfortable being honest with your doctor, consider finding someone new (and try to set up a consultation call in advance so you can ask questions and see if your new doctor is a good fit before your first visit). Keep in mind that you have more control over your health than you may have thought. Individuals play a huge role in achieving and maintaining health. If you don't have the option of finding a provider you really love, it will still make a huge difference to talk to your peers—either online or in person—and develop your own support system.

TREATMENT OPTIONS

As with many health conditions, the best treatment for fibromyalgia will depend on the individual. At times, it may take some trial and error before you discover which treatment, or combination of treatments, will work best for you. The healing process is a journey that will require patience and persistence. These are some treatment options that may be beneficial for those suffering from fibromyalgia. If you have not already, be sure to consult your medical doctor first to confirm or disprove the presence of any coexisting conditions that require medical treatment.

Acupuncture: Acupuncture is a form of traditional Chinese medicine that uses needles to stimulate certain areas of the body. It can reduce pain, inflammation, and stress associated with fibromyalgia.

Aromatherapy: This involves the use of essential oils from plants to promote healing. The essences can be inhaled or applied to the skin.

Biofeedback: Biofeedback involves sensors that monitor physiological processes like heart rate, muscle tension, and skin temperature. Visual or audio cues are then used to help individuals learn how to control their bodies and alleviate their muscle tension with their thoughts.

Chiropractic: Chiropractic adjustments remove subluxations (misalignments in the spine) that could cause nerve interference and impair function throughout the body. Some people have reported experiencing pain relief, increased energy levels, improved digestion, or even less anxiety with regular care.

Cognitive behavioral therapy: This is a type of targeted, goal-oriented psychotherapy that helps change patterns of thinking and behavior. Fibromyalgia can be triggered by trauma, and changing negative patterns will be an essential part of the healing process.

Hydrotherapy: Hydrotherapy is the use of water at varying temperatures and pressures to facilitate the healing process.

Massage therapy: Although some people with fibromyalgia do not tolerate deep tissue massage due to muscular pain and tenderness, others find relief after releasing tension with massage therapy.

Medication: Medical doctors can prescribe different types of drugs to help alleviate pain, depression, anxiety, and the inability to sleep.

Myofascial release therapy: This is a type of massage therapy that uses gentle manual pressure focused on the myofascial tissues, which are tough membranes that support your muscles.

Orthomolecular nutrition: This is the use of high-dose supplementation to achieve or maintain optimal health.

Physical therapy: This can help with relieving pain and stiffness. A physical therapist will also teach you how to improve strength and flexibility with different exercises and stretches.

An Overview of Popular Medications and Supplements

The following is a list of drugs that medical providers might prescribe for fibromyalgia, along with some of their more common side effects. You may notice that many are antidepressants. As you can tell from the name, antidepressants weren't specifically designed to treat physical pain, but for some people with conditions including fibromyalgia, arthritis, nerve damage from diabetes, and migraines, they provide pain relief. The way that antidepressants work on pain is not fully understood, but it might be related to increasing neurotransmitters in the spinal cord and thus reducing pain signals. Tricyclics are the most common type of antidepressant prescribed for pain, but some people prefer serotonin-norepinephrine reuptake inhibitors (SNRIs) or selective serotonin reuptake inhibitors (SSRIs), which typically have fewer side effects.

Drug Name	Therapeutic Effect	Common Side Effects	Drug Type
Acetaminophen	Pain relief	Liver damage	Analgesic; can be purchased over the counter; not as effective with fibromyalgia pain
Aspirin	Pain relief	Heart attack, stroke, ulcers, bleeding in the stomach or intestines	NSAID; can be purchased over the counter; not as effective with fibromyalgia pain
Celexa	Lessens pain	Decreased sex drive, fatigue	SSRI antidepressant
Cymbalta	Treats depression, anxiety, sleep issues, nerve and muscle pain	Nausea, dry mouth, fatigue, constipation, decrease in appetite, sweating	SNRI antidepressant
Elavil	Relieves pain and fatigue, improves sleep	Nausea, fatigue, dry mouth, blurred vision, constipation, change in appetite	Tricyclic antidepressant
Flexeril	Lessens pain and fatigue, improves sleep	Dry mouth, dizziness, blurry vision	Muscle relaxant

Drug Name	Therapeutic Effect	Common Side Effects	Drug Type
Ibuprofen	Pain relief	Heart attack, stroke, ulcers, bleeding in the stomach or intestines	Nonsteroidal anti-inflammatory drug (NSAID); can be purchased over the counter; not as effective with fibromyalgia pain
Lexapro	Lessens pain and depression	Decreased sex drive, impotence, insomnia, nausea, constipation, weight changes, anxiety	SSRI antidepressant
Luvox	Lessens pain and depression	Dry mouth, depressed mood, anxiety, nausea, vomiting, diarrhea	SSRI antidepressant
Lyrica	Lessens pain and fatigue, improves sleep	Sleepiness, dizziness, blurred vision, weight gain, difficulty focusing, swelling in the hands and feet, dry mouth	Nerve-related pain and anti-seizure medication

Drug Name	Therapeutic Effect	Common Side Effects	Drug Type
Naproxen	Pain relief	Heart attack, stroke, ulcers, bleeding in the stomach or intestines	NSAID; can be purchased over the counter; not as effective with fibromyalgia pain
Neurontin	Relieves pain and fatigue, improves sleep	Blurry vision, dizziness, drowsiness, weight gain, swelling in hands and feet	Pain and anti-seizure medication
Paxil	Lessens pain and depression	Headache, upset stomach, vision changes, pain, anxiety, nervousness, insomnia, strange dreams	SSRI antidepressant
Prozac	Lessens pain and depression	Headache, upset stomach, vision changes, pain, anxiety, nervousness, insomnia, strange dreams	SSRI antidepressant
Savella	Lessens pain	Nausea, constipation, dizziness, insomnia, sweating, vomiting, heart palpitations or higher heart rate, dry mouth, high blood pressure	SNRI, although it is not used to treat depression

Drug Name	Therapeutic Effect	Common Side Effects	Drug Type
Tramadol	Pain relief	Stomach pain, constipation, trouble concentrating, nausea	Narcotic; can be addictive
Zanaflex	Eases pain, fatigue, and tenderness; improves sleep	Headaches, chest pain, nausea, fever	Muscle relaxant
Zoloft	Lessens pain and depression	Decreased libido, dizziness, insomnia, fatigue, loose stools, diarrhea	SSRI antidepressant

Note:

The side effects listed are not complete. You may experience no side effects or side effects not stated here.

SUPPLEMENTS COMMONLY RECOMMENDED BY NATUROPATHS

Category	Supplement	Therapeutic Effects	Notes
Antioxidants	Beta-carotene	Fights cell damage, increases energy production	
	Vitamin C	Regulates immune function, fights cell damage, and increases energy production	Buffered vitamin C is best for anyone suffering from gastric issues
	Vitamin E		
	Coenzyme Q10	Increases energy production, protects from fights cell damage, reduces inflammation, improves heart function	
	Alpha-lipoic acid	Fights cell damage, increases energy production, reduces inflammation, and improves metabolism	
Vitamins and minerals	B-complex vitamins	Reduces pain, numbness, tingling, anxiety, and fatigue	Methylated vitamin B complex is best
	Vitamin D3	Relieves pain and fatigue	

Category	Supplement	Therapeutic Effects	Notes
	Magnesium malate	Relieve pain, fatigue, and restless legs	
Amino acids	L-theanine	Improves sleep, relaxation, and cognitive function	May interact with drugs and other supplements
	5-Hydroxytryptophan (5-HTP)	Relieves pain and depression, improves sleep	Has several drug interactions
Essential fatty acids	Flaxseed oil	Eases pain and fatigue, protects against cell damage	
	Borage oil	Reduces inflammation, pain	
	Fish oil	Eases pain and fatigue, protects against cell damage	
	Black currant seed oil	Eases pain and fatigue, protects against cell damage, reduces toxicity, improves immunity	

Category	Supplement	Therapeutic Effects	Notes
	Eicosatetraenoic acid (EPA)	Eases pain and fatigue, protects against cell damage	
	Primrose oil	Eases pain and fatigue, protects against cell damage	
Herbs	Turmeric	Reduces pain, dizziness, paresthesia, and cramps	
	Jamaican dogwood	Relieves muscle pain, spasms, anxiety attacks, headaches, neuralgias, and spasms; improves sleep	Has several drug interactions
	Devil's claw	Relieves arthritic and muscle pain	
	White willow	Eases pain	Do not use if allergic to aspirin
	Passionflower	Alleviates tension, stress, anxiety, and insomnia	Has several drug interactions
	Valerian	Alleviates tension, stress, anxiety, and insomnia	Has several drug interactions

Category	Supplement	Therapeutic Effects	Notes
	Hops	Alleviates tension, stress, anxiety, and insomnia	Has several drug interactions
	St. John's wort	Can relieve depression, anxiety, and insomnia	Has several drug interactions
	Panax ginseng	Reduces pain, increases energy, improves sleep	
Multivitamins and nutrients	Metagenics Fibroplex	Relieves pain and fatigue	Easier to find online
	Source Naturals Fibro-Response	Eases pain and fatigue	Easier to find online
	Olympian Labs Fibro X	Eases pain and fatigue	Easier to find online
	Fibro-Ease Multi	Eases pain and fatigue	Easier to find online
Others	Full Life Reuma-Art	Relieves pain	
	Cannabinoid oil	Relieves pain and anxiety, improves sleep	
	Melatonin	Improves sleep	

Category	Supplement	Therapeutic Effects	Notes
	D-ribose	Reduces fatigue	
	S-Adenosyl methionine (SAMe)	Relieves pain and depression, improves sleep	May have drug/herb interactions
	Proteolytic enzymes	Relieves pain, improves digestion and nutrient absorption	

Note:

Quality is important when it comes to supplementation. Refrain from buying supplements at pharmacies or big chains like GNC and Walmart. It is best to shop at your local health-food store or online. Check the Resources section (page 146) for recommendations on where to find supplements.

Keep in mind that several natural supplements can be contraindicated with certain medications. Do not discontinue or begin any supplements or drugs discussed in this book without first discussing it with your healthcare provider and confirming it is safe for you. These charts provide a brief summary of therapeutic effects and side effects. It is not all-inclusive.

CHAPTER 2
THE ROAD TO LASTING RELIEF

Having a clear plan for treating fibromyalgia will set you on the road to success. The goal of this book is to provide practical and easy plans based on a holistic approach to healing that you can customize based on your needs. This removes the stress and fear of not knowing what to do or where to begin. This chapter explains the different aspects of the plans and why they are a necessary part of your journey to lasting relief.

MANAGING FIBROMYALGIA ON MULTIPLE FRONTS

The body is an organism made up of many systems that work together. When one system is not functioning optimally, it will affect the other systems as well. When the body develops chronic conditions, many of its systems may experience varying levels of dysfunction. Symptoms are the body's way of letting us know that it is attempting to solve a problem. With fibromyalgia, each person can experience different symptoms, or coexisting conditions, at different intensities. Several factors likely led to the development of the dysfunction(s) causing the symptoms. According to the *Handbook of Clinical Neurology*, fibromyalgia is a very complex condition, and it requires a multidisciplinary approach in which patient self-management is key.

The next few chapters will discuss a variety of options that you can incorporate into your lifestyle to find relief. The recommendations in this book will be focused on improving emotional health, digestion, and physical movement. These are the three most important areas in achieving or maintaining health for all of us, especially those of us dealing with chronic illness. You can customize the plans in this book according to your energy levels, pain levels, and schedule. To maximize your chances of success, try to be in tune with your body's responses to the changes you make while applying these plans. The better you know your body, the better you will be able to take care of it and advocate for it.

Keep in mind that nothing in this book should be a substitute for advice you were given by your medical provider. The book is meant to be used in conjunction with the medical care you are receiving, after you have discussed it with your healthcare provider. Confirm with your healthcare provider that your lifestyle changes will not affect any established treatment regimen or any other health conditions you may have.

An Invitation to
Trust Your Inner Wisdom

Many sufferers of fibromyalgia become emotionally distressed due to others dismissing their hardship and being unsupportive. Only you know what it is like living in your body, but some people will diminish problems they cannot "see." Your frustration can actually fuel your determination to find relief. Think of this as an opportunity to see which people in your life will be most helpful in your healing process, as they will be much more willing to listen to your needs and feelings. Furthermore, cultivating self-awareness and trusting it over the opinions of others is sometimes the only path forward for many people.

Because we are all so unique, healing your body will involve trusting that your body can and will communicate with you as you pay attention to all the cues that it gives. What works for one person may or may not work for you. The journey to healing can be slow and intimidating. Success will depend on your persistence in being your biggest advocate and cheerleader, even when no one else seems to understand or believe you. Your body will communicate to you what things are helping or hindering its ability to heal. Trust me, it wasn't until I learned to understand the cues my body was giving me that I began to see progress, and this is the same pattern I see in my consultations. With practice, this will become easier over time.

THE HEALING JOURNEY, ONE STEP AT A TIME

To help you feel less overwhelmed, the fibromyalgia healing journey is broken down into different steps in order of priority.

Prioritize Rest and Emotional Health

Our bodies require rest to regenerate and recover from stress. A lack of rest or a lack of restful sleep can undermine all the hard work of maintaining a health-conscious lifestyle. Negative thoughts and emotions will also stand in the way of your success. According to Dr. Herbert Benson, author of *The Relaxation Response,* negative thinking leads to an increase in the stress hormones produced by the body, which impedes the body's ability to heal itself. Dawson Church explains in his book *The Genie in Your Genes* that our minds and behaviors can influence genetic expression. By changing our thoughts, we can truly change our lives. Our motivation, choices, and actions all begin as a thought. What's more, if you're stuck in a vicious cycle of obsessive negative thoughts directed toward yourself, you're less likely to be proactive about your health.

Restore Healthy Digestion

The food we consume becomes the building blocks for all the cells of our bodies. The ability to digest and absorb the foods we consume is what provides fuel for all of your body systems. By increasing the amount of whole foods you are eating, you improve digestion, the quality of all your cells, and their ability to function effectively. Processed foods and added sugars can increase the inflammation in our bodies and can thereby increase pain in anyone who suffers from a chronic pain condition. Improving digestion and following an anti-inflammatory diet can reduce the symptoms associated with fibromyalgia. The meal plans included in this book will be very easy to prepare. They require a minimal amount of work and can be prepared in large quantities so that you do not have to cook daily or several times each day.

Improve Physical Movement

Exercise and physical movement are crucial to anyone seeking to achieve or maintain health. Moving your body can increase energy, reduce stress, and improve mood, sleep, and cognitive function. The right type of physical movement is important to build strength and flexibility. This reduces the risk of injury and stiffness, builds muscle, and protects bones. Luckily the movement necessary to receive all these health benefits does not require strenuous workouts and can be handled in a very gentle way.

Addressing Coexisting Health Conditions

Although the focus of this book does not include a clear plan on how to address all the possible coexisting health conditions related to fibromyalgia, it is important that these conditions are not ignored. Addressing these will be part of the process to heal your body. If you are already aware of other conditions that you have, make sure you discuss with your healthcare provider what, if any, limitations they may cause. If you haven't been diagnosed with any other conditions, but something discussed in this book seems familiar, be sure to bring that to your doctor's attention so that they can confirm whether or not you have any other health conditions.

Survival Guide: "Resources Are Tight Right Now"

Living with fibromyalgia is draining. It's important to plan ahead to prevent wasting time, money, or energy on something unproductive. Before starting this plan, research available resources in your area that can help reduce costs. Write down what you find so you can refer back to it later.

Look into the following money-savers:

- Food pantries for groceries
- Coupons for items you regularly purchase
- Free or sliding-scale clinics for people without insurance
- Clearance items
- Online shopping
- Cheaper alternatives for phones, car insurance, or medical insurance with the same coverage

Save time and conserve energy with the following tactics:

- Keep a priority list of all your tasks and eliminate things that are unnecessary or detrimental to your health.
- Plan to do tasks that require the most energy at the times you are usually less fatigued, keeping in mind not to do too much.
- Reduce your workload as much as possible. Accept help when it's offered.

- Check for drive-up or delivery options at your local department stores.
- Carpool whenever possible.
- Do strenuous tasks during the day. Leave your evenings open for rest and relaxation.

CELEBRATE PROGRESS, NOT PERFECTION

The great thing about natural healing is that it does not require perfection. This frees us of the guilt of maybe not doing more on some days or doing too much on others. If you do the right thing most of the time, that is good enough. With this book, you will learn many things that you can start incorporating into your life to jump-start your natural healing process. Every time you apply something new, that is progress! Every time you experience relief from any of your symptoms, that is also progress. An easy way to prevent unnecessary frustrations is by setting realistic goals. The goal is incremental progress—not perfection.

As you are evaluating your progress, remember that everyone heals at a different pace. You probably wanted relief *yesterday*, but your actual time line may be slower. Be gentle with yourself. When we are sick and tired of being sick, we have a tendency to be our own worst enemies. Chapter 3 will explain how to avoid this in more detail.

The only way to fail is to do nothing. Any progress is a victory, and every day that you did not give up is a victory.

Keeping track of your symptoms is a great strategy to find out what treatments are working best for you. Use the following chart to keep track of what you're trying and how your body responds. Mark the corresponding day, and list the

Symptom	Scoring Criteria	Treatment Tried	Days								
			1	2	3	4	5	6	7	8	9
Pain	0 - None 10 - Extreme										
Stiffness	0 - None 10 - Extreme										
Fatigue	0 - None 10 - Extreme										
Brain Fog	0 - None 10 - Extreme										
Stress	0 - None 10 - Extreme										
Difficulty Doing Everyday Activities	0 - Fully Functional 10 - Unable to function										
Mood	0 - Happy, Calm 10 - Depressed, Anxious										
Sleep	0 - Great 10 - None										
Other _____	0 - None 10 - Extreme										
Other _____	0 - None 10 - Extreme										
Other _____	0 - None 10 - Extreme										

Remember to try new treatments one at a time, introducing new treatments after three or more days. This way, if you happen to have an adverse reaction to something, you have a clearer idea of which treatment caused it and you can discontinue it right away.

treatments you're trying that day and score your symptoms on a scale from 0 to 10, with 0 representing no problems or difficulties and 10 representing extreme problems or difficulties. Ideally, your scores will gradually become lower as your treatments progress.

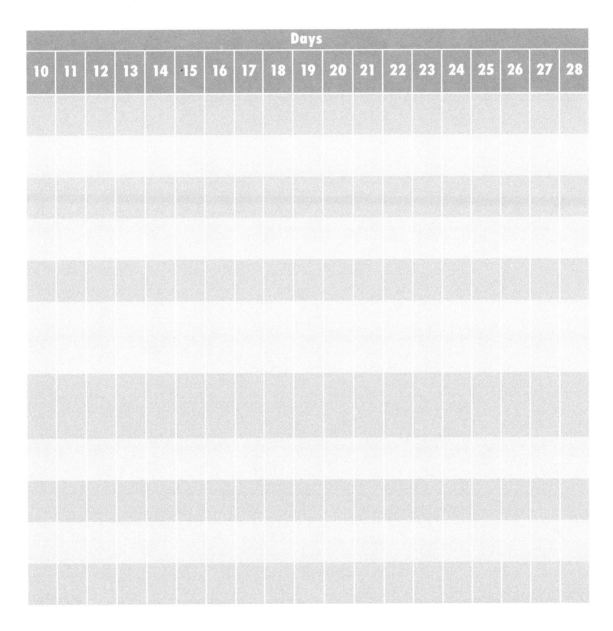

Days																		
10	11	12	13	14	15	16	17	18	19	20	21	22	23	24	25	26	27	28

CHAPTER 3
FOUR WEEKS TO SUPPORT REST AND EMOTIONAL HEALTH

Finally, you made it to your first monthly plan! This month's goal will be to get some rest and treat yourself with lots of love and kindness. You'll harness the mind-body connection and reflect on how our thoughts, emotions, and actions affect our bodies. First, we'll go over why all this matters, and then we'll get right into some strategies you can start trying out to determine which would be the most helpful for you.

HARNESS THE MIND-BODY CONNECTION

In chapter 1, we discussed the stress response and how that may cause or aggravate some of the symptoms associated with fibromyalgia. It is important to know that we can fight the stress response by learning how to activate our relaxation response. You can do this through stimulating the vagus nerve. The vagus nerve, also known as "the wanderer," is one of 12 paired cranial nerves. On each side of your body, the vagus nerve runs from the base of the brain down through your chest and into the abdomen. It sends information about the state of your organs to your brain, and it regulates muscles involved in speaking, as well as muscles in your digestive system, heart, and lungs. The nerve is responsible for your heart rate—whether that's a fast heart rate responding to danger or stress, or a slower, relaxed heart rate.

The easiest way to activate your relaxation response is almost too easy: breathe slowly and deeply. Try to exhale for longer than you inhale. Slow deep breaths will prompt the vagus nerve to slow your heart rate and cause your body to relax. Going through the motions of being calm can actually make us feel calm! Because the muscles around our vocal cords are stimulated by the vagus nerve, things like gargling, singing, and humming can also stimulate the vagus nerve. Doing other relaxing things like meditating with deep breaths, getting a massage, or doing certain types of yoga (breathing-focused Sudarshan Kriya Yoga in particular) will also stimulate the vagus nerve and facilitate your healing.

STRATEGIES FOR INCREASED RELAXATION

Now that you know more about the relaxation response, here are several strategies you can try:

Schedule a time for you. Pick a time where you can detach from other responsibilities and electronic devices. Dedicate yourself to relaxing.

Find ways to be touched. When we receive friendly touch, pressure receptors under the skin send a signal to the brain via—you guessed it—the vagus nerve, which controls the body's heart rate. Friendly touch also causes our bodies to release oxytocin, the "cuddle hormone" that plays a role in social bonding. This type of touch can come from all kinds of interactions, including hugs, kisses, holding hands, massage, or sex.

Use aromatherapy. Try essential oils like lavender, ylang-ylang, cedarwood, vetiver, bergamot, sandalwood, or chamomile in a diffuser or bath, or look for scented candles.

Listen to relaxing sounds. Find whatever is calming to you, whether it be jazz, pop music, or nature sounds like light rain.

Get creative. Doing arts and crafts can help take your focus off stress. Painting, coloring, sketching, and scrapbooking are just a few of many art forms you can try.

Picture your happy place. Visualizing something you find pleasant can be a valuable part of your relaxation practice. Find whatever works for you. Maybe it's a waterfall or a garden. You could also try focusing on a sweet moment in your life that gives you a cozy feeling.

Move your body. Try certain types of exercise like yoga or tai chi. These are great at reducing pain and anxiety in people with fibromyalgia. This will be discussed further in chapter 5.

Meditate or pray. Different types of meditation and prayer can activate the relaxation response and promote healing. Meditation involves calming yourself, typically by focusing on an object, a thought, or a visualization. Detailed steps for a meditation are included under the Remedies for Relaxation section on page 41.

Breathe slowly and deeply. As previously discussed, slow deep breaths will stimulate the vagus nerve and relax your body. It may be a good idea to try this throughout the day, whenever you catch yourself stressed, anxious, or tense.

Have fun. You may enjoy watching funny movies, reading a book, interacting with animals, or even playing a board game with a friend. Any activity that brings you laughter and happiness can help you relax.

RESTORING DEEP, NOURISHING SLEEP

Rest is vital for our health and a huge part of our lives. The average person spends about one-third of their time asleep. Sleep makes it possible for our brains to work properly. We need it to maintain pathways in our brain that allow us to learn, form memories, and concentrate. Healthy sleep has two basic types: rapid eye movement sleep, or REM, and non-REM sleep that happens in three stages. We cycle in and out of these sleep phases, and our brain waves and neurons behave differently during each phase. Healthy sleep is integral to the function of your whole body, especially your brain, heart, lungs, metabolism, and immune system. Researchers have found that a lack of sleep increases a person's risk of disorders, including depression and diabetes. If you are having difficulty falling asleep at night, try to evaluate your sleep hygiene.

Here are several tips to help improve your sleep hygiene and increase deep sleep:

Set a time for sleep and getting out of bed. We have a biological clock that regulates several bodily functions, including sleep, and it is very responsive to routine. Try to go to bed and get out of bed at the same time each day.

Make your bedroom into a sleep haven. Try to stay away from your bedroom if you are not going to sleep. Don't have a TV or a computer in your bedroom. Your body should begin to associate the room with relaxation.

Avoid electronic devices altogether for an hour before bedtime. The blue light from these devices (including TVs, smartphones, computers, and tablets) disrupts melatonin production, which is a hormone our bodies naturally produce in the absence of light to make us sleepy.

Set the climate in your room. It is best to keep the bedroom dark, cool, and quiet. If you find soft music, white noise, or nature sounds relaxing, try playing those.

Avoid stimulating activity before bedtime. For two to three hours before your designated bedtime, don't exercise and, if you can, stay away from anything that stresses you out, including big discussions or arguments with family or friends, work, and the news. Instead, focus on practicing your relaxation techniques.

Avoid eating and drinking. Your dinner should be no later than two hours before your bedtime, and it should be the lightest meal of the day. Drinking too many liquids close to bed or drinking caffeine and alcohol can also disrupt sleep.

Remove clocks from your bedroom. Staring at a clock when you cannot sleep only creates more anxiety. Remove any clocks that you can see from your bed.

Avoid taking naps. If you have insomnia and only get sleep in the early afternoon, a short 30-minute nap can be helpful, but avoid naps close to your bedtime.

Address any anxiety before bedtime. Try any of the relaxation techniques mentioned or the supplements mentioned in chapter 2 on page 14, like L-theanine. Additionally, sometimes we obsess over things we are trying to ignore, so writing them down in a journal can calm your mind and allow you to move on.

Address any sleep disorders. If sleep apnea or restless leg syndrome is keeping you up at night, be sure to address this with your healthcare provider.

Survival Guide: "I Just Can't Sleep!"

Having suffered from insomnia for almost ten years, I completely understand that some days, despite all efforts, you just won't fall asleep. If this is what you are experiencing, the worst thing you can do is stay in bed stewing in frustration as you try to force yourself to sleep. After 20 minutes of lying in bed, it is best to get out of bed and focus on relaxing. Read a book, listen to soft music, write a poem, meditate—do whatever works for you. When you start to feel sleepy, you can go back to bed. This is a good time to make sure you are not stuck in a negative thought pattern. Do not assume that you will never be able to sleep or make catastrophic projections about your future ("I can't sleep. I will never get healthy. I won't be able to function tomorrow"). The reality is that most people have difficulty with sleep at some point in their life, and this can be regulated with time. You are not alone. Set a realistic goal: Just focus on relaxing and resting as much as possible until sleep comes.

THE CRITICAL IMPORTANCE OF SELF-COMPASSION

Early in my journey with fibromyalgia, I was in a constant battle with my inner critic. I could not turn off that harsh, judgmental voice. Before I developed the condition, I considered myself to be a very rational, logical, level-headed person. I thought anxiety and depression happened to "other types of people." Then I became one of those people. I felt trapped in a self-destructive mind that would obsess over things that I knew I had no control over. It was a long battle of self-blame and self-disgust, which eventually led to a spiritual and emotional breakthrough. Part of my healing process was learning to address the root cause of all these negative thought patterns.

Humans are social creatures, and we are all born hardwired to give and receive love. Somewhere along the way, we receive imperfect love, and it creates wounds that lead to negative thought patterns and behaviors. These wounds also affect our perceptions and set the foundation for emotional health issues. Self-compassion is one of the ways we can begin to break free from it.

Self-compassion is a decision to be understanding and kind with ourselves through hard times and failures. When the brain performs and receives acts of kindness, it releases some of the same feel-good hormones we get from physical touch, like endorphins and oxytocin. When we are kind to ourselves, the brain can receive it in the same way it would an act of kindness from someone else. Thus, self-compassion is the most reliable source of kindness during difficult times. In this way, being kind to ourselves can reduce stress, anxiety, and depression; in turn, it can increase immunity and enhance the healing process. According to Dr. Kristin Neff, a psychology professor and the author of *Self-Compassion*, there are three core components that make up this practice.

"THE THREE ELEMENTS"

The three core components of self-compassion are being kind to ourselves, recognizing common humanity, and practicing mindfulness.

Self-kindness involves being understanding of ourselves instead of falling into self-judgment and self-criticism. Keep in mind that this does not mean we ignore our flaws, weaknesses, and imperfections. It does mean that we try to talk to ourselves as we would talk to a dear friend: with love and understanding.

The second component, recognizing common humanity, requires that we acknowledge that all of our flaws are part of the human experience, and we can be gentle with ourselves. When we fail, we don't belittle ourselves; we remember that *everyone fails sometimes*. This also stops us from isolating our issues or feeling that our pains are exceptional, that only we feel this particular hurt. We are never alone.

Finally, practicing mindfulness requires introspection and staying in the present moment—the only place where change is possible, since the past is already over and the future has not yet begun. This is where we get in touch with reality and become aware of our negative thoughts, emotions, and actions as they are, without exaggerating or minimizing. When we are mindful, we are fully aware of where we are, where we want to go, and how we can go about getting there. Awareness sets a path for success. This is why mindfulness and self-compassion are so crucial for our health.

At the end of this chapter you will find several exercises to assist you with practicing these three elements of self-compassion.

YOUR 28-DAY REST AND EMOTIONAL HEALTH PLAN

Now you are ready to prepare your first monthly plan where your focus will be getting rest and improving your emotional health. Before you get started, take some time to evaluate your situation and your daily routines. Can you think about what can be removed from your schedule to make time for getting sleep and staying grounded? Once you have visualized how you will fit this into your day, you can begin to fill out the plan for this first month. In order to fill out this plan you will need to:

- Select realistic times to go to bed and wake up each day that allow you at least seven hours of sleep or rest.
- Choose three things from the relaxation remedies and emotional health practices listed on pages 41 through 63 that you will do each day for the next seven days. Each week you may select three different things to try. At least one of the three things you incorporate into your routine must be an emotional health practice.
- Commit to a relaxing 30-minute routine before going to bed and list on the worksheet what you will be doing to relax during this time. This routine can include any of the three relaxation remedies and emotional health practices you've chosen to do each day for seven days. It just needs to be consistent.
- Complete the Tracking Symptoms, Treatments, and Results worksheet from chapter 2 (pages 28 and 29) at the end of each day so that you can track your progress. If you notice progress with any of the remedies or practices you have selected, you can continue doing them the following week.

Write the name of each practice or remedy you plan to try in the blank spaces for each week (refer to the lists on pages 41 through 63 for examples). For your bedtime routine, write the list of things you plan to do. And if there's a practice you know works for you, you can reuse it in a subsequent week, too.

	Emotional Health Practice #1	Practice or Remedy #2	Practice or Remedy #3	30-Minute Bedtime Routine
Week 1				
Week 2				
Week 3				
Week 4				

REMEDIES
FOR RELAXATION

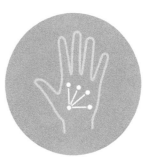

ACUPRESSURE

There are several acupressure points that can be used for reducing stress, pain, fatigue, and anxiety. Finding these points and applying light pressure or massaging for a three to five minutes can help you relax and prepare for bed. (You can try this throughout the day, if you want.) Try out any of the acupressure points on the following pages.

YINTANG

This point is located between the eyebrows and can reduce anxiety and provide relief for headaches, nasal congestion, and insomnia.

Instructions

1. Locate the point as shown in the image.

2. Gently press the point with your finger or massage in slow circles.

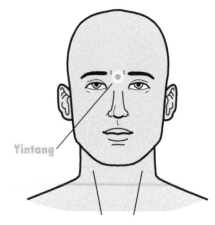

REN 17 (SHANZHONG)

This point is located in the center of the breastbone, in the fourth space between the ribs. It can be beneficial for relaxation, heart health, and asthma.

Instructions

1. Locate the point as shown in the image.

2. Gently press the point with your finger or massage in small circles for about 3 to 5 minutes.

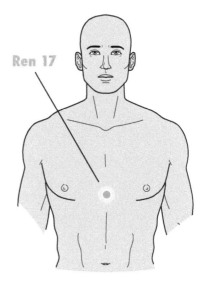

SHEN MEN

This point is located in the center, upper portion of your ears. This point can be beneficial for relaxation, reducing inflammation, and overall wellness.

Instructions

1. Locate the point as shown in the image.

2. Lightly pinch the point with your index finger and thumb or massage in a circular motion for one minute.

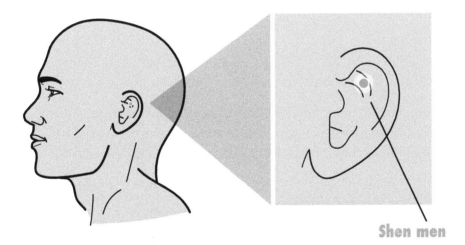

Shen men

AROMATHERAPY BATH

This remedy combines the healing properties of aromatherapy and hydrotherapy. The warm bathwater is good for relaxing and decreasing pain levels, and the essential oil selected for the bath can further enhance relaxation.

Required Ingredients

- Coconut oil
- Epsom salt
- Essential oil

Required Equipment

- Bathtub

Instructions

1. Fill up your tub with warm water.

2. Choose an essential oil that is good for relaxation: lavender, ylang-ylang, chamomile, sandalwood, cedarwood, or any others mentioned in this chapter if they are not contraindicated with any medication you are on.

3. Mix about 10 to 15 drops of your essential oil with half a cup of Epsom salt and two teaspoons of coconut oil.

4. Add the mixture to your bathwater.

5. Soak in the bath for about 20 minutes or more. Enjoy.

Tip: If you do not have a bathtub or you are having a flare-up and find it too difficult to get in and out of a tub, you can try purchasing soap with a calming scent or running a diffuser with some of these essential oils in your bathroom while you take a hot shower.

PROGRESSIVE MUSCULAR RELAXATION

When muscles are initially tensed, they can relax more deeply. In this practice, you actively tense specific muscles for 10 seconds and then relax them for a few seconds, progressing throughout the body until your entire body is fully relaxed. Doing this exercise before bed can help relieve any tension in the muscles.

Instructions

1. **Lie down in a relaxed position.** Find a quiet, calm place where you can do this exercise without distractions or interruptions. Keep your legs slightly apart and your arms at your sides. Close your eyes and allow your weight to sink into the bed or recliner.

2. **Tense and relax your toes.** Curl your toes and tense them as much as possible. Hold for 10 seconds, then relax your toes. Take a slow deep breath and feel your toes relax further as you exhale.

3. **Continue to tense parts of your body for 10 seconds, then relax as you exhale.** Move on to your feet and calves, then your thighs and buttocks. Tense your abdominal muscles as if you were drawing your belly button into your spine. Relax. Tense your hands, then relax.

4. **Tense your biceps.** Bring your arms to your shoulders, hold for 10 seconds, then relax.

5. **Tense your triceps.** Tighten the back of your arms, hold for 10 seconds, then relax.

6. **Shrug your shoulders hard.** Hold for 10 seconds, then relax.

7. **Arch your back.** Hold for 10 seconds, then exhale.

8. **Take a deep breath and tighten your chest muscles.** Hold for 10 seconds, then relax.

9. **Push your head back and tense your neck.** Hold for 10 seconds, then relax.

10. **Bring your chin to your chest and tense your neck.** Hold for 10 seconds, then relax. Look to the right and tense your neck. Hold for 10 seconds, then relax. Look to the left and repeat.

11. **Open your mouth as wide as you can.** Tense the muscles around your mouth. Hold for 10 seconds, then relax your mouth.

12. **Squeeze your eyes shut as hard as you can.** Hold for 10 seconds, then relax.

13. **Raise your eyebrows and scrunch your forehead as hard as you can.** Hold for 10 seconds, then relax.

14. **Take a slow deep breath.** Feel your entire body relax as you exhale.

Tip: Remember you are only tensing one area of your body at a time while the rest remains relaxed. You can repeat the exercise in any area that still feels tense. There are plenty of videos on YouTube that can guide you through this exercise so you don't have to stop and read instructions as you go along. Personally, I would not find that very relaxing!

REFLEXOLOGY MASSAGE

There is nothing like a good foot massage before bed. Here is a simple procedure for giving yourself a reflexology massage. You can also use this as a guide for a friend or significant other.

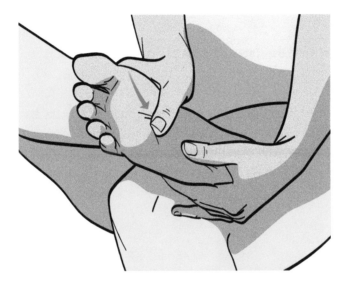

Instructions

1. Pick a foot and place your hands on the sides of that foot. Press into the sides of your foot in a circular motion with both hands for 10 seconds. Reverse directions and continue gently pressing the sides of your foot.

2. Turn your foot so you're looking at the sole. Cup your foot with both hands and place your thumbs on the soles of your feet. Press gently into your foot in a circular motion, repeating a few times.

3. Press into each of your toes with your fingers, first clockwise and then counterclockwise.

4. Press into your ankles with your hands, first clockwise and then counterclockwise.

5. Use a thumb walk through the solar plexus area in the ball of the foot, as shown on the image on page 47.

6. Next, apply pressure to the head and neck reflex sites at the base of your toes by pinching with your fingers and holding for about 15 seconds.

7. Move on to press any other areas you feel you may need to relieve tension in.

8. Then finish by repeating steps 2 through 7 to relax your foot.

9. Repeat the process on the other foot.

Tip: You can also use one drop of your preferred essential oil—try lavender or sandalwood if you're unsure—and mix it with a tablespoon of coconut oil or jojoba oil and use this as part of your foot massage.

RELAXING TEA

Teas are a great way to receive the healing benefits of herbs. Warm tea before bed can be very relaxing and even help with sleep. Chamomile, lavender, and lemon tea bags are great options, and they're available at most grocery stores. Valerian root may be particularly good at easing people into sleep; it is available in some grocery stores but might be more readily available in a health-food store. As you drink your tea, filter out distractions. Try to focus on the smell of the tea, the warmth, the taste. Feel free to sweeten with a teaspoon of honey if you wish.

Tip: Remember that some herbs may interact with medications. There is a link in the Resources section (page 146) where you can check for drug-herb interactions, but if you are not sure, it is best to confirm with your healthcare provider before trying herbal teas if you are taking medication.

STRESS-REDUCING BREATHS

Slow deep breathing is a very simple relaxation technique. You can do it anywhere, anytime, and it can help center you even if you only take a few breaths.

Instructions

1. Inhale slowly through your nose for at least four seconds. Your abdomen should expand when you inhale.

2. Exhale slowly through your mouth for four to eight seconds. Your abdomen should return to normal.

3. Take at least three deep breaths. You can deep-breathe for as long as 15 minutes if you are able to.

Tip: If you catch yourself feeling overwhelmed, anxious, or stressed at any time, take a quick break and work on your deep breaths.

WRITING

Writing can be therapeutic and reduce stress and anxiety, thereby improving relaxation, sleep, and healing. Writing down our thoughts or troubles can be a way of releasing them. It is often easier to express ourselves on paper, especially when we know no one will be reading what we write.

Required Equipment

- Paper
- Pencil or pen

Instructions

1. Find a calm, quiet place with few distractions.

2. Take a minute to think about what has been on your mind that day.

3. Once you've given it some thought, write about whatever you want to. If you are unsure where to start, try writing about how your day went, how you are feeling, and why you think you are feeling that way.

Tip: If you have difficulty writing out your thoughts, try making a gratitude list. Make a list of everything and everyone you are grateful for and why. Think about these people or experiences as you get ready to go to bed.

MEDITATION

Meditation is a great way to relax the body and focus the mind. The processing and/or perception of pain can be reduced during meditation. Practice meditating so you can return to it when you have heightened levels of pain.

Instructions

1. Decide what will be the focal point in your meditation: your breath, an object in the room, an image, a word, or part of a scripture.

2. Find a place with no distractions where you can sit comfortably.

3. Set a timer for at least five minutes.

4. Begin to take slow deep breaths.

5. Focus your attention on the breaths.

6. Scan your body and try to release any tense muscles.

7. Direct your attention or thoughts to the focal point you chose.

8. If you catch yourself wandering, bring yourself back to focus.

Tip: If five minutes is too difficult at first, do not force it. It's okay to struggle! Try to meditate for as long as you can. With practice, you can make small improvements over time.

GUIDED IMAGERY

This exercise is very similar to meditation. With guided imagery, you focus your thoughts on a place or image that creates positive feelings; this redirects you from negative thoughts. You can do this in any position you find comfortable.

Instructions

1. Find a quiet place.

2. Choose the position that is most comfortable to you and close your eyes.

3. Take slow deep breaths.

4. Start to picture a place that makes you feel very calm or safe.

5. Focus your thoughts on this place: Is it warm? What sounds do you hear? What do you feel?

6. Keep your thoughts on this place for a few minutes or until you feel relaxed.

Tip: If imagining or remembering the place is too difficult, find a picture that you can look at instead to focus on. It can even be a piece of art in your home that you find very relaxing.

EMOTIONAL FREEDOM TECHNIQUE

Like acupuncture, this technique focuses on restoring balance to the body's energy. Tapping the meridian points shown in the image can help reduce stress or negative emotions.

Instructions

1. Focus on a fear or problem.

2. Rate the intensity of your discomfort from 0 to 10.

3. Tell yourself that you accept yourself, even with the fear or problem. For example, if I were concerned that I was falling behind on work, I could say, "Even though I am falling behind on work, I deeply and completely accept myself."

4. Begin by tapping the KC point in the image while repeating your phrase three times.

5. Then tap the remaining points—first TOH, then EB, then SE, then UE, then UN, then CH, then CB, then UA— about five times each using two or more fingers.

6. As you tap, recite a short phrase to remind yourself of the issue you are having. For example, "too much work."

7. Rate your intensity again, and, if you are not at 0, you can repeat the process.

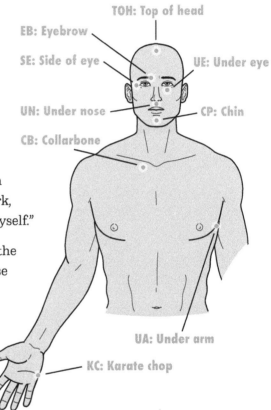

TOH: Top of head

EB: Eyebrow

SE: Side of eye

UE: Under eye

UN: Under nose

CP: Chin

CB: Collarbone

UA: Under arm

KC: Karate chop

EMOTIONAL HEALTH PRACTICES

EMOTIONAL AWARENESS JOURNALING

Our thoughts are the root of our emotions and our actions. Negative thinking prevents us from reaching our potential, and journaling is an excellent way to process our thoughts and let go of negativity. This exercise can be done whenever you catch yourself stuck in negative thinking. You can also try it before your bedtime if negative thinking is making it difficult to fall asleep.

Instructions

1. Take your time and write down the negative thoughts you are experiencing. (Example: **My family does not care about me.**)

2. Write down the facts. (Example: **My family hasn't called me all week. I wish they would call me.**)

3. Now write down the interpretation of the facts. Why did this cause negative thoughts? (Example: **I think that they don't call me because they don't care about me.**)

4. Review the facts. Choose an alternate interpretation focusing on what you know to be true. (Example: **It is possible that they are busy or having their own problems. I could reach out to them.**)

5. Write down the new thoughts or emotions this new interpretation creates and read them out loud. (Example: **My family has not called me, but they still love and care for me. Let me call them to make sure they are okay and tell them I miss them.**)

Tip: At times it can be very difficult to re-evaluate our interpretation of events. Often that is why we got stuck in negative thinking in the first place: It's hard to see things from different perspectives. If you find yourself stuck, try to imagine you are counseling a close friend, a child, or another loved one. If your friend were in your shoes, what would you say to comfort your friend?

GET RID OF ANTS

The psychiatrist Daniel Amen writes about ANTs—automatic negative thoughts—in his book *Change Your Brain, Change Your Life*. These ANTs affect your mood, behavior, and physical health. They can consist of:

- **Thinking in extremes or absolutes:** Thoughts with words like *always, never, everyone, no one,* and *every time.*
- **Mind reading:** Believing you know what the other person is thinking without them telling you their thoughts.
- **Fortune-telling:** Predicting the worst possible outcome in a situation.
- **Personalizing:** Assuming others' bad behavior is your fault.
- **Labeling:** Attaching a negative label to yourself or others.
- **Blaming:** Blaming others for your problems or actions.
- **Focusing on the negative:** Only thinking about the negative aspect of someone or a situation.
- **Thinking with your feelings:** Believing in your feelings without questioning them.
- **Guilt beating:** Thinking with words like *I have to, I must, I should have* or *shouldn't have.*

Instructions

1. Write down your ANT on a piece of paper.

2. Note what type of ANT it is from the list above.

3. Counter the ANT with a rational interpretation of the situation.

Example:

Thought: I *have to* clean the entire house and visit my mom today.

Type of ANT: Guilt beating.

Counter: I want to clean the entire house and visit my mom. I can choose to do that if I feel well enough, or I can choose not to and rest.

RECITE AFFIRMATIONS DAILY

We can purposefully change the cycle of negative thoughts by reciting positive affirmations, out loud, several times a day. This is an easy way to start reprogramming your mind and transforming your life! Your affirmations must be unique to you.

Instructions

1. Think about or write down some of the negative thoughts you are struggling with.

2. Write down an affirmation that counters each thought. For example, if my negative thought is *I am tired of being unhealthy and my life sucks*, my affirmation could be *I have the power to make changes in my life*.

3. Place your list of affirmations in an area of your house that you will see frequently.

4. Read your affirmations **out loud** each time you see them, at least three times daily. Return to them when you find yourself stuck in negative thinking.

Tip: The Emotional Awareness Journaling exercise (page 54) can be useful in coming up with affirmations if you are having difficulty thinking of any. You can also turn to the internet for affirmations.

TREAT YOURSELF AS YOU'D WANT YOUR LOVED ONE TO BE TREATED

We are usually much better at giving advice than we are at applying it. When we are upset with our situation, it affects our ability to think rationally.

Instructions

1. When you find yourself overwhelmed with a situation or beating yourself up, think of a close friend, a loved one, or a child you care for in that situation. You are likely much more compassionate with them than you are with yourself.

2. Ask yourself the following questions: "What would I do or say to that individual? What advice would I give? How would I treat that person?"

3. Take some time to evaluate how you have been treating yourself and responding to your situation and how you think your friend or loved one would feel or respond if you responded that way to them.

4. Try treating yourself the way you would treat your loved one and follow the advice you would give them.

IDENTIFY AND COMMUNICATE PRIMARY EMOTIONS

Anger is another possibly toxic emotion that can stand in the way of our healing. A healthy anger fuels us so that we can resolve an issue or stand up against injustice. Unhealthy anger leads to abusive behavior toward yourself or others, and it can turn into bitterness and resentment. Addressing the emotions that lead to your anger is part of self-love and self-compassion.

Instructions

1. When you feel angry as a result of an event or situation, commit to taking a break. This may mean physically separating yourself from the people involved in the conflict if possible, or ending a conversation or discussion that has resulted in your anger.

2. Take this time to think about what resulted in the anger. Are you feeling frustrated, scared, ashamed, disappointed, humiliated, insecure, or rejected? Accept these feelings as part of your humanity.

3. Next, think about what expectation you had that was broken to cause these hurt feelings. Were these expectations realistic? Is there a "should" statement behind these expectations? Where did these expectations come from? Do others involved in the conflict have the same expectations of themselves as you have of them?

4. Identify and counter any ANTs that may have led to the anger.

5. When you have finished this time of introspection, you can return to the situation by communicating your primary emotions and expectations, instead of voicing any ANTs.

Tip: It may help to journal this process, as writing helps most of us process our information more effectively. If the conflict arises with someone you are in a relationship with, you can share this exercise with them and see if both of you can commit to using this to de-escalate anger when resolving conflict.

JUST SAY NO

Being a people-pleaser can be draining. People-pleasing can seem like an expression of love and generosity, but it can actually stem from a need for approval from others. Sometimes, putting our own needs second is a way that we show a lack of love to ourselves. Part of being kind to ourselves is creating healthy boundaries so that we are able to help ourselves first and help others when we are well enough to do so.

Instructions

1. Reflect on recent situations where you may have done too much or put up with too much. Did you clean the house during a flare-up? Did you go to a birthday party when you hadn't slept at all the previous night?

2. Write out some boundaries that you can stick to, prioritizing your physical and emotional health.

3. Set boundaries based on your physical capacities. These may vary daily based on energy and pain levels. Commit to your daily relaxation time with no interruptions (except for emergencies, of course).

4. Set boundaries against any and all toxic conflict behavior which will increase stress hormones. No one should be yelling at you, for example. You do not have to tolerate it.

5. Be clear and loving in communicating these boundaries to your friends and loved ones.

Tip: Domestic abuse is about power. Chronic illness can make people more vulnerable to skewed power dynamics and abusive relationships. No one has the right to abuse you. If you are regularly suffering emotional abuse, financial abuse, or violence at home, please try to get help right away. The National Domestic Violence Hotline is a great place to start. Their number is 1-800-799-7233. You can also try contacting a local domestic violence shelter, or a Legal Aid practice if you need an attorney.

FORGIVE YOURSELF AND FORGIVE OTHERS

Forgiveness is another way that we practice self-compassion. When we forgive ourselves, we are acknowledging that we have done something wrong and we are choosing to be kind to ourselves because making mistakes is part of the human condition. If you find yourself troubled by guilt, then this journaling exercise is for you.

Required Equipment

* Journal
* Pencil or pen

Instructions

1. Grab a journal and write down some of the things you are feeling guilty about.

2. If you notice any ANTs in your thought process, correct those first. (For example: **I am a horrible spouse.** Counter: **I was not kind to my partner today.**)

3. If necessary, give yourself a reality check. You are only responsible for your actions, so if any guilt is coming from anyone else's actions, write and then read aloud the following statements from Dr. Norman Wise's book *Succeeding at Life*:

   · I am not responsible for anyone else's actions.
   · Each of us can choose to do right or wrong.
   · No one can force another person to make a choice.
   · I can influence a choice, but the person still has to make the choice.

4. For any guilt resulting from your actions, write down an acknowledgment of the wrong. (For example: **I made the choice to yell at my spouse.**)

5. Next, write down a compassionate response to your wrong action. (For example: **I can choose to forgive myself for making the wrong choice. I can choose to forgive my spouse if they responded unkindly. I can choose not to yell at my spouse again. I can choose to acknowledge my wrongdoing to my spouse, take responsibility, and ask for forgiveness.**)

6. Read your compassionate responses out loud.

YOU ARE NOT ALONE

Loneliness isn't always rational. You could be surrounded by friends and still experience loneliness; it is a response to *perceived* isolation that is not necessarily always based in reality. Loneliness can feel out of our control, but it is something we have the power to address.

Instructions

1. Evaluate how much you are interacting with others. Are you feeling lonely because you're not getting enough interaction, or because you're not feeling a significant connection with any of the people you interact with?

2. Write down and address any ANTs that may be associated with your loneliness.

3. If you have people in your life whom you would like to connect with more deeply, try to create that connection.

    - If you have unresolved conflict in a relationship, seek counseling or therapy.
    - Try finding common interests that you can share together. Dedicate time to enjoying these things together.

4. If you are feeling unsupported or misunderstood because of your condition, try connecting with a local support group. I have provided a web address in the Resources section (page 146) to help you find the fibromyalgia support group nearest you.

REJECTION ISSUES

Abandonment, or perceived abandonment, is another trauma that can leave us with emotional issues. We can develop abandonment issues after a range of circumstances, including the loss of a parent through death or actual abandonment, bad parenting, bullying, or a painful breakup. Here are some steps you can take to start addressing any rejection issues.

Instructions

1. Write down your earliest childhood memories of rejection.

2. Acknowledge your feelings associated with the rejection: maybe you feel fear, anger, grief, or something else. Write down what you feel.

3. Acknowledge these as normal feelings. There is nothing wrong with you for feeling this way.

4. Tell yourself that you are not to blame for the rejection.

5. Avoid only thinking about the positive aspects of whoever rejected or abandoned you. Example: a parent who left may not have been fit to take good care of you.

6. Write down and meditate on the following statements:

   - Rejection is not my fault.
   - I am not responsible for people's inability to love me as I am.
   - I am imperfect, flawed, **AND LOVABLE**.

7. Think about the triggers that bring up your fear of rejection. Maybe conflict, criticism, or pursuing relationships stirs those old fears for you? Write down your triggers.

8. Write down statements to address these fears. If your triggers are conflict and criticism, for example, you could write down something like this: "Conflict is a normal part of relationships. Conflict does not make me unlovable. Criticism is a form of feedback, and it is necessary for growth. I can accept when I am wrong, reject false criticism, and still

be lovable. Another person's decision to reject or abandon me is not my fault, and there is nothing I can do to control it."

Tip: Recite the statements under step 6 aloud daily. Refer back to this exercise whenever your rejection issues are triggered by a current situation.

FEAR / ANXIETY

Anxiety may have biological, psychological, and/or spiritual causes. Certain hormonal or neurotransmitter imbalances, as well as nutritional deficiencies, can cause severe anxiety and fear. Anxiety can also be a response to childhood trauma or stem from the need to have control over situations that you cannot control. It can even be due to a crisis of faith. Anxiety is a normal part of the human experience, and being aware and kind to yourself will help you along the path to overcoming it.

Instructions

1. Acknowledge and accept that you are anxious or fearful.

2. Be kind to yourself. Remind yourself that **everyone experiences fear and anxiety at times, and many people suffer from it on a regular basis. You are not alone.**

3. Meditate on the possible causes. Remind yourself that anxiety is a normal, human response.

4. Identify and counter ANTs associated with your anxiety.

5. Consider whether a lack of understanding may be causing the anxiety. Are you scared of something because you do not understand it? Are you anxious because you don't know what lies ahead? If so, use some of your free time to read about the object of your fears or worries.

6. Seek help from your healthcare provider. If you have chronic anxiety or a phobia, you may need help from an expert in that field.

CHAPTER 4
FOUR WEEKS TO RESTORE HEALTHY DIGESTION

After addressing any emotional health issues, the next step is to improve digestion. This month's goal is to restore your digestion with proper nutrition so that each meal is simple, nourishing, and, hopefully, easy to digest. You can continue the remedies and practices from last month's plan, or you can focus only on nutrition this month.

THE ROLE OF FOOD IN FIBROMYALGIA

There are several known trigger foods that can cause fibromyalgia pain for anyone, but food allergies or sensitivities that are unique and specific to the individual may also cause digestive issues. Eliminating my own trigger foods was what gave me the most relief from fibromyalgia pain. My sensitivities were so strong that I did not even have to eat the foods—just chopping trigger foods or being near them while they were being chopped was enough to cause a flare-up and set me back for several days.

There are some foods that we should all try to avoid, whether we have chronic pain or not. These include sugar, refined carbohydrates, fried foods, artificial sweeteners, and processed foods containing food coloring, preservatives, and other additives. Basically, if you look at the package a food comes in and see a very long list of ingredients, it's very processed, and you should try to avoid that food (especially if the ingredients are unpronounceable!).

Other foods are more specific to inflammation. To minimize inflammation, you should try to avoid wheat and other high-gluten grains, corn, soy, dairy, nightshade vegetables (peppers, tomatoes, eggplant, potatoes), citrus, beef, pork, shellfish, eggs, trans fats, processed oils, processed sugar, artificial sweeteners, caffeine, alcohol, and peanuts. For some people, even eggs can trigger inflammation. For others, a range of fruits, vegetables, additives, and dairy products high in fermentable oligosaccharides, disaccharides, monosaccharides, and polyols (shortened to FODMAPs) are a trigger. These foods can cause digestive issues, respiratory issues, skin issues, emotional or psychological issues, weight issues, and pain.

Luckily, there are also plenty of foods that have healing anti-inflammatory effects. These foods include most fruits and vegetables, whole grains, nuts, seeds, fish, and many spices. When it comes to proper nutrition, the key is quality. Fresh organic produce is preferred. If that is not possible, make sure to wash your produce thoroughly. Whole grains, as opposed to refined grains, have a higher content of fiber and micronutrients needed to sustain health. Fish, particularly the kinds with lower mercury levels, like herring or haddock, are best when they are wild-caught. If you eat poultry, you should try to find meat that's been pasture-raised, is free of antibiotics and added hormones, and was not fed corn or gluten. Because there is no dietary fiber in fish and poultry, they should be combined with fiber-rich vegetables for optimal digestion.

DIETARY GUIDELINES FOR MANAGING FIBROMYALGIA

Here are some general guidelines for the foods and beverages you put into your body:

Stay hydrated. For adults, up to 60 percent of our bodies are made of water. Water lubricates our joints, flushes waste from our bodies, regulates our temperature through sweating, and is the building block of every cell. Make sure you drink plenty of water! It is generally best to sip water throughout the day instead of trying to drink large amounts at once.

Eat more raw fruits and vegetables. Our diet should be mostly plant-based. Consuming large quantities of meat, especially processed meat, has been linked to an increased risk for cancer and heart disease, among other conditions. When we cook food, it can lose some of its nutritional value. If you don't have any digestive issues where it may be contraindicated, enjoy an abundance of raw fruits and vegetables, including green leafy vegetables, several times a day.

Enjoy fresh vegetable juices. Fiber is great for our health and gut microbiome. Adding vegetable juices will increase the absorption of micronutrients and enzymes, adding more nourishment to your health-conscious diet. A well-nourished body is properly equipped to heal itself. I recommend not adding fruit juices, except for lemon or green apple, to avoid causing a spike in blood sugar levels.

Enjoy healthy fats. The omega-3 fatty acids found in foods like fish, flaxseed, chia seeds, and walnuts reduce inflammatory responses in the body. People need omega-3s— eicosapentaenoic acid (EPA), docosahexaenoic acid (DHA), and alpha-linolenic acid (ALA)—as part of a healthy diet because they form parts of cell membranes. These fats can help ease the symptoms of chronic inflammatory conditions:

Spice up your meals. There are many herbs and spices that have anti-inflammatory properties, including ginger, cumin, rosemary, clove, thyme, oregano, cinnamon, anise, and turmeric (particularly in combination with black pepper). They can be used to season foods, and many can be consumed as a tea.

Diversity is best. Each food is filled with different combinations of nutrients. Having a diverse diet is a great way to improve your nutrition.

Avoid triggers. As previously discussed, you should avoid processed foods and junk food, and of course, avoid foods you are personally sensitive to. Because these foods will create an inflammatory response in the body, it will be impossible to completely heal without avoiding them as much as possible. The recipes in this book emphasize a diet made up of nutritious whole foods free from common fibromyalgia trigger foods.

Supplement as needed. Unfortunately, when the body is not well, it usually needs more nutrients than we can realistically consume with foods alone, and supplementation will be a necessary part of correcting deficiencies. Probiotics and/or prebiotics may also be necessary to ensure you have the right population of gut microbes for healthy digestion and immunity.

FOODS TO AVOID, MODERATE, AND ENJOY

Common Food Groups	Avoid	Moderate (0–3x Weekly)	Enjoy
Fruits and Vegetables	Potatoes, tomatoes, eggplants, bell peppers, chili peppers, cayenne pepper		All non-nightshade vegetables, starchy roots, fresh or frozen fruits
Grains	Refined grains such as white rice, bread, and white flours; gluten-rich foods such as wheat, barley, and rye		Gluten-free carbs like brown rice, quinoa, amaranth, and buckwheat
Legumes*	Canned legumes that have added salts		Beans (kidney, lima, pinto, black), lentils and peas (pigeon peas, split peas)
Healthy Fats	Peanuts or peanut butter, canola oil, or cooking with any oil except for coconut oil, olive oil, or avocado oil		Nuts and seeds such as almonds, walnuts, pumpkin seeds, and sunflower seeds

Common Food Groups	Avoid	Moderate (0–3x Weekly)	Enjoy
Fish and Seafood	Shellfish and crustaceans such as crab, oysters, lobster, snails, shrimp, clams, and shark	Fish such as salmon, sardines, haddock, cod, mackerel, herring, flounder, and pollock	
Poultry and Eggs*		Organic, cage-free, no hormones or antibiotics	
Meat	Beef, pork, lamb, deli meats, and processed meats like sausage and hotdogs	Soy-based foods and meat alternatives like tofu and tempeh	
Beverages	Carbonated beverages, alcohol, caffeinated beverages, cow milk, juices with added sugars or fructose	Fresh-pressed vegetable juices, non-dairy milks	Water, water infused with fruits or vegetables, non-caffeinated herbal teas

Common Food Groups	Avoid	Moderate (0–3x Weekly)	Enjoy
Sweeteners	White sugar, brown sugar, artificial sweeteners		Honey, maple syrup, stevia
Spices and Condiments	Paprika, margarine, barbecue sauce, condiments containing added sugar, high-fructose corn syrup, and MSG	Mustard, mayonnaise, non-dairy butter	All dried herbs, sea salt, vinegars, spices, liquid aminos, nutritional yeast
Others	Fast foods, candy, desserts	Non-dairy cheese, dark chocolate	

*These foods may be triggers for some people with fibromyalgia, especially if they also suffer from irritable bowel syndrome. If you notice significant pain or digestive upset including abdominal pain, bloating, and gas after eating these foods, you may need to remove them as well.

THE ELIMINATION DIET

Because food sensitivities are fairly common among people with fibromyalgia, it is very important to identify any food sensitivities you may have. It is possible that not all of the common triggers are triggers for you, and it is also possible that you have other triggers not mentioned in this book. It's important to note that food sensitivities can shift over time. To find out what types of foods make you most comfortable—and most uncomfortable—you can try an elimination diet.

An elimination diet is broken into two different stages: elimination and reintroduction. During the elimination phase, you remove any suspected trigger foods from your diet for three to four weeks. I recommend that you eliminate the foods in the "avoid" column in the charts on pages 69 through 72, as well as some of the foods that are known for being common trigger foods. In a full elimination diet, all "avoid" foods are eliminated at once. Some people find that it may be too difficult and overwhelming. If this is the case, you can do a partial elimination diet where you remove a few of the suspected triggers. If you start to feel better during the elimination phase, then you may have already found some of your trigger foods. If not, you may need to do another round of the elimination diet until you find your triggers.

REINTRODUCING FOODS TO IDENTIFY TRIGGERS

It is very important that you reintroduce the possible trigger foods properly so that you can accurately determine whether or not each is a trigger food. Here is a list of the steps you can take while reintroducing foods:

- After at least 21 days of eliminating the suspected trigger foods, you can begin reintroducing them.
- Introduce the foods one at a time as you watch for symptoms. Eat the suspected trigger food at least twice a day for three days.

- If you felt better during the elimination phase, then you probably have a good idea of what symptoms may be returning when you reintroduce a trigger food. Some of these common symptoms are headaches, joint pain, bloating, fatigue, stomach pains, difficulty sleeping, and skin issues.
- If the symptoms do not return when introducing a food for three days, you can move on to introduce another food until you find your trigger.
- If your symptoms do return, then you have found a trigger! Eliminate this food from your diet, and when the symptoms subside again, you can move on to try another suspected trigger to see if it is also a trigger.
- Once you have positively identified any triggers, you will have a much better idea of which foods are best for you.

Food sensitivities can go away with time. You can try to reintroduce some of your trigger foods after six months of avoiding them. Reintroduce them one at a time to find out if you have overcome your sensitivities. However, remember that some of the foods you eliminated were probably not very nutritious foods, regardless of whether or not they are trigger foods. You should still try to avoid those, even if they don't seem to trigger symptoms.

The thought of cooking can be overwhelming, especially when you're dealing with pain and fatigue (and the possibly daunting prospect of changing your diet). Here are a few tips that may help:

Prepare meals in advance. Take advantage of days you are well enough to prepare meals in bulk. These meals can be refrigerated or frozen for later. Then on days when you are not feeling your best, all you have to do is warm up the food.

Look for recipes. Making changes to your diet can be very stressful. When I learned all the foods that I had to stop and start eating, I felt like I had to learn to cook all over again. What helped me was looking for recipes online that met my requirements. Luckily, this book provides several recipes to get you started.

Simplify the cooking. You can buy frozen fruits and vegetables, or prechopped ingredients. There are even some whole grains that come in a box and only need to be microwaved. Using a slow cooker, where you don't have to keep an eye on the food, could be helpful.

YOUR 28-DAY MEAL PLAN

Your plan this month involves creating an anti-inflammatory meal plan. You have several easy and nutritious recipes to choose from that meet the general dietary guidelines for fibromyalgia. Most recipes contain no more than five ingredients, excluding sea salt, black pepper, oil, and lemon juice. All the ingredients are affordable, and most of them require minimal work. For example, using dried herbs and frozen produce generally means you don't have to wash, peel, or chop anything. The snacks will not require any recipes at all—you'll munch on fruit, non-dairy yogurt, or nuts, which means less work for you. The meal recipes can be prepared in big enough quantities so that you can eat from them up to three times. If you make larger quantities and store them in the fridge or freezer, that means you won't need to prepare more than seven recipes for an entire week's worth of meals. As you proceed, make sure to do the following:

- When you look over the recipes, check for any foods that you are allergic to or suspect may be a trigger food. If so, avoid these recipes, or use a quick and easy anti-inflammatory substitute for that ingredient.
- Create a 28-day meal plan that includes three meals and a snack for each day.
- Remember to fill out your Tracking Symptoms, Treatments, and Progress worksheet found on pages 28 and 29 at the end of each day to keep a log of any improvements or flare-ups you experience with this plan.

This meal plan is for one person. In most cases, the servings will be used later in the week. A few additional servings are not accounted for on the meal plan. If you have leftovers, you can eat them throughout the week as snacks in between meals.

Week 1

For this week, there will be extra servings of the following meals. These can be eaten as snacks or added to a meal for a little more bulk if needed.

- Mediterranean Chickpea Salad (1 serving)
- Vegetable and Quinoa Coconut Stew (2 servings)

Week 1	Breakfast	Lunch	Dinner
Monday	Baked Oatmeal (page 91)	Mediterranean Chickpea Salad (page 97)	Vegetable and Quinoa Coconut Stew (page 93)
Tuesday	Sweet Potato Toasts with Fried Egg (page 88)	Leftover Vegetable and Quinoa Coconut Stew	Sheet Pan Salmon, Asparagus, and Butternut Squash (page 105)
Wednesday	Leftover Baked Oatmeal	Leftover Mediterranean Chickpea Salad	Leftover Vegetable and Quinoa Coconut Stew
Thursday	Leftover Sweet Potato Toasts with Fried Egg	Leftover Vegetable and Quinoa Coconut Stew	Leftover Sheet Pan Salmon, Asparagus, and Butternut Squash
Friday	Leftover Baked Oatmeal	Leftover Mediterranean Chickpea Salad	Slow Cooker White Chicken Chili (page 108)
Saturday	Tofu Vegetable Scramble (page 87)	Leftover Slow Cooker White Chicken Chili	Tofu and Brown Rice Salad (page 101)
Sunday	Leftover Tofu Vegetable Scramble	Leftover Tofu and Brown Rice Salad	Leftover Slow Cooker White Chicken Chili

Recipe Plan

1/2 recipe Baked Oatmeal

1/2 recipe Sweet Potato Toasts with Fried Egg

1 recipe Tofu Vegetable Scramble

1 recipe Mediterranean Chickpea Salad

1 recipe Vegetable and Quinoa Coconut Stew

1/2 recipe Sheet Pan Salmon, Asparagus, and Butternut Squash

1/2 recipe Slow Cooker White Chicken Chili

1/2 recipe Tofu and Brown Rice Salad

Week 2

For this week, there will be an additional serving of the following meals. These can be eaten as snacks or added to a meal for a little more bulk if needed.

- Brown Rice Salad Bowl (1 serving)
- Creamy Lentil Carrot Soup (2 servings)

Week 2	Breakfast	Lunch	Dinner
Monday	Brown Rice Salad Bowl (page 89)	Avocado Tuna Salad Wraps (page 104)	Stuffed Baked Sweet Potatoes (page 95)
Tuesday	Sweet Potato Toasts with Fried Egg (page 88)	Leftover Avocado Tuna Salad Wraps	One-Pot Chicken, Beans, and Greens (page 107)
Wednesday	Leftover Brown Rice Salad Bowl	Leftover Stuffed Baked Sweet Potatoes	Creamy Lentil Carrot Soup (page 94)
Thursday	Leftover Sweet Potato Toasts with Fried Egg	Leftover Creamy Lentil Carrot Soup	Leftover One-Pot Chicken, Beans, and Greens
Friday	Leftover Brown Rice Salad Bowl	Leftover Creamy Lentil Carrot Soup	Leftover Stuffed Baked Sweet Potatoes
Saturday	Spinach and Mushroom Omelet (page 90)	Leftover Stuffed Baked Sweet Potatoes	Leftover One-Pot Chicken, Beans, and Greens
Sunday	Baked Oatmeal (page 91)	Leftover One-Pot Chicken, Beans, and Greens	Leftover Creamy Lentil Carrot Soup

Recipe Plan
1 recipe Brown Rice Salad Bowl
½ recipe Sweet Potato Toasts with Fried Egg
½ recipe Spinach and Mushroom Omelet
1 recipe Baked Oatmeal (leftovers are used in the meal plan for week 3)
1 recipe Avocado Tuna Salad Wraps
1 recipe Stuffed Baked Sweet Potatoes
1 recipe One-Pot Chicken, Beans, and Greens
1 recipe Creamy Lentil Carrot Soup

Week 3

For this week, there will be an additional serving of the following meals. These can be eaten as snacks or added to a meal for a little more bulk if needed.

- Chicken Zucchini Noodle Soup (1 serving)
- Slow Cooker White Chicken Chili (1 serving)

Week 3	Breakfast	Lunch	Dinner
Monday	Leftover Baked Oatmeal (from week 2)	Chickpea and Brown Rice Bowl (page 99)	Chard and Tofu Stir-Fry over Lentils (page 96)
Tuesday	Sweet Potato Toasts with Fried Egg (page 88)	Leftover Chard and Tofu Stir-Fry over Lentils	Chicken Zucchini Noodle Soup (page 106)
Wednesday	Leftover Baked Oatmeal (from week 2)	Leftover Chickpea and Brown Rice Bowl	Leftover Chard and Tofu Stir-Fry over Lentils
Thursday	Leftover Sweet Potato Toasts with Fried Egg	Leftover Chicken Zucchini Noodle Soup	Vegetable and Quinoa Coconut Stew (page 93)
Friday	Leftover Baked Oatmeal (from week 2)	Leftover Chard and Tofu Stir-Fry over Lentils	Slow Cooker White Chicken Chili (page 108)
Saturday	Spinach and Mushroom Omelet (page 90)	Leftover Chicken Zucchini Noodle Soup	Leftover Vegetable and Quinoa Coconut Stew
Sunday	Leftover Spinach and Mushroom Omelet	Leftover Vegetable and Quinoa Coconut Stew	Leftover Slow Cooker White Chicken Chili

Recipe Plan

½ recipe Sweet Potato Toasts with Fried Egg

1 recipe Spinach and Mushroom Omelet

½ recipe Chickpea and Brown Rice Bowl

1 recipe Chard and Tofu Stir-Fry over Lentils

1 recipe Chicken Zucchini Noodle Soup

½ recipe Vegetable and Quinoa Coconut Stew

½ recipe Slow Cooker White Chicken Chili

Week 4

For this week, there will be an additional serving of the following meals. These can be eaten as snacks or added to another meal for a little more bulk if needed.

- Brown Rice Salad Bowl (1 serving)
- Amaranth and Chickpea Tabbouleh Salad (1 serving)

Week 4	Breakfast	Lunch	Dinner
Monday	Brown Rice Salad Bowl (page 89)	Avocado Tuna Salad Wraps (page 104)	Amaranth and Chickpea Tabbouleh Salad (page 100)
Tuesday	Tofu Vegetable Scramble (page 87)	Leftover Avocado Tuna Salad Wraps	Sheet Pan Salmon, Asparagus, and Butternut Squash (page 105)
Wednesday	Leftover Brown Rice Salad Bowl	Leftover Sheet Pan Salmon, Asparagus, and Butternut Squash	Leftover Amaranth and Chickpea Tabbouleh Salad
Thursday	Leftover Tofu Vegetable Scramble	Leftover Amaranth and Chickpea Tabbouleh Salad	Roasted Veggie and Buckwheat Tahini Bowl (page 102)
Friday	Leftover Brown Rice Salad Bowl	Leftover Roasted Veggie and Buckwheat Tahini Bowl	One-Pot Chicken, Beans, and Greens (page 107)
Saturday	Spinach and Mushroom Omelet (page 90)	Leftover One-Pot Chicken, Beans, and Greens	Chickpea and Brown Rice Bowl (page 99)
Sunday	Leftover Spinach and Mushroom Omelet	Leftover Chickpea and Brown Rice Bowl	Leftover One-Pot Chicken, Beans, and Greens

Recipe Plan

1 recipe Brown Rice Salad Bowl

1 recipe Tofu Vegetable Scramble

1 recipe Spinach and Mushroom Omelet

1 recipe Avocado Tuna Salad Wraps

1 recipe Amaranth and Chickpea Tabbouleh Salad

½ recipe Sheet Pan Salmon, Asparagus, and Butternut Squash

½ recipe Roasted Veggie and Buckwheat Tahini Bowl

1 recipe One-Pot Chicken, Beans, and Greens

½ recipe Chickpea and Brown Rice Bowl

TIPS AND TRICKS FOR SUCCESS

Eating on a meal plan is a great way to get introduced to healthier eating. The benefits of eating on a meal plan are that you don't have to try to figure out day by day what you are going to prepare, you know exactly what grocery items you will need since your meals have been planned in advance, and you know how to make the taste appealing to your palate. Just in case meal plans are new for you, here are a few tips on how to make the process easier:

- **Check if anyone else in your household would like to follow your meal plan.** This not only means that there won't be a need for additional meal prep, but it also means that you have possible helpers in preparing the meals.

- **Write out a specific grocery list.** Since you know exactly what you will be eating for the next month, you can create a grocery list that includes only the items that you need. This way you only purchase healthy items, and you won't have the temptation in the kitchen of going back to comfort foods that keep you from meeting your goals.

- **Purchase the right containers.** Freezer-safe storage bags may be the best option to store food. They take up less space than bowls, and you can throw them away after using them or, if you've purchased reusable freezer bags, you can rinse them out. They are generally cheaper than freezer-safe food storage containers, if you don't already have those.

- **Use frozen foods or pre-prepped ingredients.** You'd be surprised at how many healthy pre-prepped ingredients you can find at an affordable price. They may be more expensive than the usual ingredients, but in my opinion the price is worth it if it means less work while still eating healthy.
- **Invest in some helpful gadgets.** There are quite a few affordable gadgets that can help you out in the kitchen. Investing in a slow cooker, a rice cooker, or a food chopper can make the cooking process even easier.

BREAKFAST
RECIPES

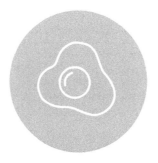

Tofu Vegetable Scramble

Tofu contains essential B vitamins. When paired with grains, it creates an easily digested protein. In this simple scramble, nutritional yeast provides a cheesy flavor and anti-inflammatory turmeric creates a beautiful yellow color. You can serve this scramble with a side of brown rice, quinoa, or a piece of gluten-free toast.

SERVES 2 / PREP TIME: 10 MINUTES / COOK TIME: 5 MINUTES

8 ounces extra-firm tofu

1 tablespoon extra-virgin olive oil

½ teaspoon ground turmeric

2 cups chopped baby spinach

2 tablespoons nutritional yeast

Salt

Black pepper

2 tablespoons chopped scallions, green parts only

1. Using several paper towels, press down on the tofu firmly to expel as much water as possible. Remove the paper towels and, using a fork, crumble the tofu into small pieces.

2. In a skillet, heat the oil over medium-high heat. Sauté the tofu and turmeric for 2 to 3 minutes until heated through.

3. Add the spinach and nutritional yeast and cook for an additional 2 minutes, until the spinach wilts.

4. Season with salt and pepper and serve topped with scallion greens.

Ingredient Tip: Leftover tofu that you don't use in the recipe can be stored in fresh water in an airtight container for up to 1 week. Drain and refresh the water every 2 days.

PER SERVING: Calories: 189; Total Fat: 14g; Sodium: 118mg; Sugars: 1g; Carbohydrates: 5g; Fiber: 1g; Protein: 14g

Sweet Potato Toasts with Fried Egg

Sweet potatoes are loaded with vitamin A precursor beta-carotene and make a bright, nutrition-packed base for your breakfast. Used like mini pieces of toast and topped with an egg, salad greens, and pesto, this is a simple and filling whole food breakfast that is easy to make happen on a busy morning.

SERVES 4 / PREP TIME: 10 MINUTES / COOK TIME: 20 MINUTES

2 large sweet potatoes, cut lengthwise into ½-inch-thick slices

1 tablespoon extra-virgin olive oil

4 large eggs

4 cups salad greens

2 tablespoons prepared pesto

1. In a toaster oven or under a broiler, toast the sweet potatoes for 12 to 15 minutes, flipping once, until just tender.

2. While the sweet potatoes are toasting, heat the oil in a skillet over medium-high heat. Crack the eggs into the skillet, keeping the yolks intact. Cook for 3 to 5 minutes, then cut the whites apart to flip each each egg. Cook for about 20 to 30 seconds longer, until the whites are just set. Carefully remove the eggs from the pan and set aside.

3. To assemble the toasts, place 1 or 2 sweet potato slices on each plate and top with 1 cup of salad greens. Place the egg on top, then top each with ½ teaspoon of pesto.

Recipe Tip: For even more flavor, use microgreens, fresh herbs, or arugula in place of the salad greens.

PER SERVING: Calories: 210; Total Fat: 13g; Sodium: 182mg; Sugars: 3g; Carbohydrates: 15g; Fiber: 3g; Protein: 9g

Brown Rice Salad Bowl

Brown rice, a whole grain with intact bran layers (unlike processed white rice), is a great source of B vitamins, making it a perfectly energizing start to your day.

SERVES 4 / PREP TIME: 5 MINUTES / COOK TIME: 35 MINUTES

1½ cups water

1 cup brown rice

3 tablespoons extra-virgin olive oil, divided

4 large eggs

2 tablespoons rice vinegar

Salt

Black pepper

4 cups arugula or salad greens

2 tablespoons chopped scallions, green parts only

1. In a small pot, combine the water and rice and bring to a boil. Reduce the heat to low, cover, and cook for 30 to 35 minutes until tender.

2. In skillet, heat 1 tablespoon of oil over medium-high heat. Crack the eggs into the skillet, keeping the yolks intact. Cook for 3 to 5 minutes, then cut the whites apart to flip each egg. Cook for about 20 to 30 seconds longer, until the whites are just set but the yolk is still runny. Carefully remove from the pan and set aside.

3. In a small bowl, whisk the remaining 2 tablespoons of oil and the vinegar and season with salt and pepper.

4. Divide the rice into individual serving bowls and top each with 1 cup of arugula. Top with a fried egg and drizzle each with 1½ teaspoons of dressing.

Recipe Tip: Brown rice is a staple that can be made in bulk to cut prep time. Make a double batch and store in the refrigerator for up to 5 days, or freeze in freezer-safe storage bags or containers for up to 3 months.

PER SERVING: Calories: 345; Total Fat: 16g; Sodium: 128mg; Sugars: 1g; Carbohydrates: 38g; Fiber: 3g; Protein: 11g

Spinach and Mushroom Omelet

Mushrooms provide a delicious, meaty flavor to vegetarian and vegan dishes. The mix of dill, Kalamata olives, and mushrooms in this simple omelet creates a deeply savory dish. You get it started on the stove, then transfer it to the oven to cut down on hands-on cook time.

SERVES 2 / PREP TIME: 10 MINUTES / COOK TIME: 22 MINUTES

4 large eggs

¼ teaspoon salt

¼ teaspoon freshly ground black pepper

1 tablespoon Onion- and Garlic-Infused Oil (page 110) or extra-virgin olive oil

4 ounces mushrooms, sliced

¼ cup chopped pitted Kalamata olives

2 tablespoons chopped dill

¼ cup chopped scallions, green parts only

1. Preheat the oven to 400°F.

2. In a large bowl, whisk the eggs, salt, and pepper.

3. In a large oven-safe skillet, heat the oil over medium-high heat. Sauté the mushrooms for 4 to 5 minutes until softened and browned.

4. Pour the eggs into the skillet and sprinkle with the olives and dill. Continue to cook for 1 to 2 minutes, until set on the bottom. Sprinkle with scallions.

5. Transfer to oven and cook for 10 to 15 minutes, until set.

Substitution Tip: Substitute other fresh herbs like parsley, cilantro, or basil for a different flavor. Adding canned or frozen artichoke hearts to the omelet makes it even heartier.

PER SERVING: Calories: 259; Total Fat: 19g; Sodium: 563mg; Sugars: 2g; Carbohydrates: 8g; Fiber: 3g; Protein: 16g

Baked Oatmeal

Baked oatmeal is a simple twist on a breakfast favorite. Baked with peaches, honey, and cinnamon, this dish is perfect to make ahead and enjoy all week. Oats are high in protein, and they're an easy way to get a filling breakfast.

SERVES 6 / PREP TIME: 10 MINUTES / COOK TIME: 40 MINUTES

2 cups rolled oats

2 tablespoons honey

2 tablespoons
extra-virgin olive oil

1 teaspoon
baking powder

1 teaspoon ground
cinnamon

½ teaspoon salt

2 cups chopped
peaches

2 cups unsweetened
almond milk

1. Preheat the oven to 350°F.

2. In a medium bowl, toss the oats, honey, oil, baking powder, cinnamon, and salt. Mix well.

3. In a baking pan, place the peaches in an even layer on the bottom. Add the oat mixture on top and press down. Pour the almond milk on top.

4. Bake for 40 minutes, until the top layer looks golden brown and the oatmeal is firm. Let cool for 10 minutes, then serve on its own or with coconut yogurt.

Variation Tip: For more protein, add 1 cup of chopped nuts to the mixture. Pecans, walnuts, and cashews are all good choices.

PER SERVING: Calories: 298; Total Fat: 9g; Sodium: 198mg; Sugars: 10g; Carbohydrates: 46g; Fiber: 7g; Protein: 10g

VEGETARIAN ENTREES

Vegetable and Quinoa Coconut Stew

In this hearty stew, quinoa and chickpeas provide the protein while coconut milk provides a rich and creamy texture, perfect for either lunch or dinner. To avoid nightshades like chile peppers that are often found in curry powder, you can make your own blend with the easy spices listed in the tip below.

SERVES 6 / PREP TIME: 10 MINUTES / COOK TIME: 20 MINUTES

2 tablespoons Onion- and Garlic-Infused Oil (page 110) or extra-virgin olive oil

1 (15-ounce) can chickpeas, drained and rinsed

6 cups water

1 cup quinoa

1 (13.5-ounce) can full-fat coconut milk

1 cup shredded carrots

1 tablespoon nightshade-free curry powder (see Tip)

Salt

Black pepper

1. In a pot, heat the oil over medium heat and sauté the chickpeas for 3 to 5 minutes, stirring regularly, until lightly browned.

2. Add the water and quinoa and simmer for 15 minutes, until the quinoa is tender.

3. Add the coconut milk, carrots, and curry powder. Season with salt and pepper and serve.

Ingredient Tip: Make your own nightshade-free curry mixture. In a small jar or container, combine 2 teaspoons of ground turmeric, 1 teaspoon of ground cumin, 1 teaspoon of ground coriander, 1 teaspoon of ground ginger, ½ teaspoon of ground mustard, and ¼ teaspoon of ground cinnamon. Store in an airtight container, in a cool location, for up to 1 month.

PER SERVING: Calories: 348; Total Fat: 21g; Sodium: 52mg; Sugars: 3g; Carbohydrates: 34g; Fiber: 6g; Protein: 9g

Creamy Lentil Carrot Soup

Lentils are a great vegetarian staple because you don't need to spend much time cooking them. Here, red lentils are used to create this delicious soup, and carrots are paired with them for added nutrition. This makes a great lunch, especially with a salad or some leftover roasted vegetables.

SERVES 6 / PREP TIME: 10 MINUTES / COOK TIME: 15 MINUTES

1 tablespoon Onion- and Garlic-Infused Oil (page 110) or extra-virgin olive oil

1 cup split red lentils, rinsed

5 cups water

3 medium carrots, roughly sliced

1 (13.5-ounce) can coconut milk

1 tablespoon nightshade-free curry powder (page 93)

Salt

Black pepper

¼ cup chopped fresh cilantro

¼ cup coconut milk yogurt

1. In a large skillet, heat the oil over medium-high heat. Add the lentils and sauté for 1 minute.

2. Add the water and carrots and bring to a simmer. Cook for about 10 minutes, until the lentils and carrots are tender.

3. Using an immersion blender, process the soup until smooth. (If you don't have an immersion blender, you can also transfer the mixture to a regular blender. Just be sure to take out the vent in the blender lid and place a cloth or paper towel over the vent. This is to let steam out of the blender so it won't get trapped and potentially burst out.)

4. Stir in the coconut milk and curry powder and heat through. Season with salt and pepper.

5. Serve topped with 1 tablespoon each of cilantro and coconut milk yogurt.

Ingredient Tip: If you can't find red lentils, you can use any other variety, but you may need to increase the cooking time. Red lentils cook very quickly and nearly disintegrate as they cook, making them a great option for a soup.

PER SERVING: Calories: 280; Total Fat: 17g; Sodium: 63mg; Sugars: 3g; Carbohydrates: 26g; Fiber: 5g; Protein: 10g

Stuffed Baked Sweet Potatoes

Loaded with broccoli and protein-rich black beans, these sweet potatoes are a nourishing vitamin- and antioxidant-rich meal that is perfect for planning ahead for meal prep. These stuffed potatoes require little hands-on time, making them fairly easy to prepare.

SERVES 4 / PREP TIME: 10 MINUTES / COOK TIME: 35 MINUTES

---

4 medium sweet
potatoes
1 (16-ounce) bag frozen
broccoli
2 tablespoons tahini
2 tablespoons Onion-
and Garlic-Infused
Oil (page 110) and
extra-virgin olive oil
Salt
Black pepper
1 (15-ounce) can
black beans, drained
and rinsed

1. Preheat the oven to 350°F.

2. Using a fork, poke each sweet potato a couple times, then wrap in aluminum foil. Place the potatoes on a baking sheet and bake for 25 to 35 minutes, until they're easily pierced with a fork.

3. Steam the broccoli according to the package directions in the microwave or on the stove.

4. In a small bowl, mix the tahini and oil until combined. Season with salt and pepper.

5. To serve, divide the black beans and broccoli on each potato, then drizzle with tahini dressing.

Ingredient Tip: Tahini is ground sesame paste. Look for it in the international section or nut butter section of your grocery store. If you can't find it, you can process sesame seeds with a mild-tasting oil in a high-speed blender until smooth.

PER SERVING: Calories: 389; Total Fat: 12g; Sodium: 139mg; Sugars: 7g; Carbohydrates: 59g; Fiber: 17g; Protein: 16g

Chard and Tofu Stir-Fry over Lentils

Lentils are a versatile protein. In this recipe, they're a bed for the tofu and chard stir-fry. Swiss chard cooks quickly, but its fibrous stems add another dimension to the dish.

SERVES 4 / PREP TIME: 10 MINUTES / COOK TIME: 20 MINUTES

4 cups water
1 cup green lentils
8 ounces firm tofu
2 tablespoons Onion- and Garlic-Infused Oil (page 110) or extra-virgin olive oil
1 pound Swiss chard, greens and stems separated and chopped
2 tablespoons tamari
Juice of 1 lime
Black pepper
Salt

1. In a large pot, combine the water, lentils, and salt, and bring to a boil. Reduce the heat to low, partially cover, and simmer for 15 to 20 minutes, until the lentils are tender.

2. Meanwhile, using several paper towels, press down on the tofu firmly to expel as much water as possible. Remove the paper towels and chop the tofu into 1-inch pieces.

3. In a large skillet, heat the oil over medium-high heat. Sauté the tofu for 3 to 4 minutes on each side, until browned. Remove and set aside.

4. Add the chard stems and sauté for 3 to 4 minutes until tender. Add the chard leaves and continue to stir until wilted. Stir in the tamari and lime juice and add the tofu back to the pan. Season with salt and pepper.

5. Serve the lentils topped with the chard and tofu mixture.

Variation Tip: Other greens work well in this dish. Collards, turnip greens, and mustard greens can add flavor and substantial nutritional value.

PER SERVING: Calories: 341; Total Fat: 12g; Sodium: 1,046mg; Sugars: 3g; Carbohydrates: 39g; Fiber: 8g; Protein: 24g

Mediterranean Chickpea Salad

Cooking with frozen vegetables is a great way to conserve your energy. For this recipe, packaged cauliflower rice (often available frozen) can be prepared in the microwave while you chop the rest of the ingredients. Chickpeas provide plenty of protein in this easy, veggie-forward salad.

SERVES 4 / PREP TIME: 10 MINUTES / COOK TIME: 5 TO 10 MINUTES

1 (16-ounce) bag cauliflower rice

1 (15-ounce) can low-sodium chickpeas, drained and rinsed

1 English cucumber, chopped

½ cup chopped pitted Kalamata olives

2 tablespoons Onion- and Garlic-Infused Oil (page 110) or extra-virgin olive oil

1 tablespoon red wine vinegar

1 teaspoon Italian seasoning

Salt

Black pepper

1. Steam the cauliflower rice according to the package directions, then set aside to cool.

2. In a large bowl, toss together the cooled cauliflower rice, chickpeas, cucumber, and Kalamata olives.

3. In a small bowl, mix the oil, vinegar, and Italian seasoning. Toss into the salad and season with salt and pepper. Serve immediately or chill for 2 to 3 hours to allow the flavors to meld.

Variation Tip: Increase the protein in this recipe by adding 8 ounces of firm tofu, drained and chopped into ½-inch pieces.

PER SERVING: Calories: 237; Total Fat: 11g; Sodium: 379mg; Sugars: 7g; Carbohydrates: 29g; Fiber: 9g; Protein: 9g

Miso Mushroom Tofu Salad

Miso, a fermented soybean paste, adds a savory flavor. Miso ranges from a creamy yellow with a milder flavor to dark amber with a stronger flavor. Any miso works in this dish.

SERVES 4 / PREP TIME: 10 MINUTES / COOK TIME: 35 MINUTES

1½ cups water
1 cup brown rice
1 (8-ounce) package firm tofu
2 tablespoons Onion- and Garlic-Infused Oil (page 110) or extra-virgin olive oil, divided
8 ounces brown mushrooms, quartered
1 tablespoon miso
4 cups arugula
Salt (optional)
Black pepper
¼ cup chopped scallions, green parts only

1. In a small pot, combine the water and rice and bring to a boil. Reduce the heat to low, cover, and cook for 30 to 35 minutes until tender.

2. Meanwhile, use several paper towels to press down on the tofu firmly to expel as much water as possible.

3. In a skillet, heat 1 tablespoon of oil over medium-high heat, and sauté the tofu and mushrooms for 4 to 5 minutes, stirring occasionally, until the tofu is lightly browned and the mushrooms are softened. Remove from the heat and set aside.

4. Meanwhile, in a small bowl, whisk the miso and remaining 1 tablespoon of oil. Stir the mixture into the tofu and mushroom mixture.

5. When the rice is done, transfer to a large bowl and toss with the tofu and mushrooms. Mix in the arugula and season with salt (if desired) and pepper. Serve topped with scallion greens.

Variation Tip: Add about 2 teaspoons of grated fresh ginger to the miso mixture for even more flavor.

PER SERVING: Calories: 266; Total Fat: 9g; Sodium: 171mg; Sugars: 2g; Carbohydrates: 41g; Fiber: 3g; Protein: 7g

Chickpea and Brown Rice Bowl

This bowl comes together quickly, using canned chickpeas as the protein source. If you make the rice in advance, you can put this together in just 10 minutes. Chickpeas are rich in protein and fiber, which, along with brown rice, will keep you fuller for longer.

SERVES 4 / PREP TIME: 10 MINUTES / COOK TIME: 35 MINUTES

1½ cups water

1 cup brown rice

1 cup coconut milk yogurt

1 tablespoon Onion- and Garlic-Infused Oil (page 110)

½ teaspoon ground cumin

Salt

1 (15-ounce) can chickpeas, drained and rinsed

1 cucumber, chopped into bite-size pieces

1. In a small pot, combine the water and rice and bring to a boil. Reduce the heat to low, cover, and cook for 30 to 35 minutes until tender. Fluff with a fork and let cool for about 10 minutes.

2. In a small bowl, mix the yogurt, oil, and cumin. Season with salt.

3. Place the rice into individual serving bowls. Top with the chickpeas and cucumber. Drizzle each bowl with dressing and serve.

Variation Tip: Add 1 cup of any type of salad greens to the bowl to add more fiber and increase your vegetable consumption.

PER SERVING: Calories: 357; Total Fat: 9g; Sodium: 223mg; Sugars: 5g; Carbohydrates: 61g; Fiber: 8g; Protein: 10g

Amaranth and Chickpea Tabbouleh Salad

Amaranth is high in protein. In this salad, it is combined with bright lemon and the nutritional powerhouse parsley. With high levels of vitamins A and C as well as iron, this is one herb that can be used generously in your cooking.

SERVES 4 / PREP TIME: 10 MINUTES / COOK TIME: 20 MINUTES, PLUS 2 HOURS TO CHILL

2 cups water

1 cup amaranth

1 large cucumber

1 (15-ounce) can low-sodium chickpeas, drained and rinsed

1 cup chopped fresh parsley

¼ cup chopped pitted Kalamata olives

2 tablespoons freshly squeezed lemon juice

1 teaspoon grated lemon zest

1 tablespoon extra-virgin olive oil

Salt

Black pepper

1. In a small pot, bring the water and amaranth to a simmer. Reduce the heat, cover, and continue to simmer for 20 minutes, until the amaranth is fluffy and the water is absorbed. Set aside and let cool.

2. In a large bowl, toss the cooled amaranth, cucumber, chickpeas, parsley, olives, lemon juice, lemon zest, and oil. Season with salt and pepper. Cover and refrigerate for 2 to 3 hours to chill and allow the flavors to combine. Serve.

Variation Tip: Pine nuts are fun to add to this salad for a little crunch. You can also try adding a handful of finely chopped romaine lettuce to each bowl when serving.

PER SERVING: Calories: 312; Total Fat: 10g; Sodium: 225mg; Sugars: 5g; Carbohydrates: 48g; Fiber: 8g; Protein: 12g

Tofu and Brown Rice Salad

Ginger helps boost circulation and makes an excellent flavor addition to a wide range of dishes. In this salad, ginger ties the flavors together along with tamari, for a quick and nutritious salad.

SERVES 4 / PREP TIME: 10 MINUTES / COOK TIME: 35 MINUTES

1½ cups water
1 cup brown rice
8 ounces firm tofu
2 tablespoons Onion- and Garlic-Infused Oil (page 110) or extra-virgin olive oil, divided
2 tablespoons tamari, divided
1-inch piece ginger, peeled and minced
1 cup shredded carrot
3 scallions, green parts only, finely chopped

1. In a small pot, combine the water and rice and bring to a boil. Reduce the heat to low, cover, and cook for 30 to 35 minutes until tender.

2. Using several paper towels, press down on the tofu firmly to expel as much water as possible. Remove the paper towels and cut the tofu into 1-inch cubes.

3. In a skillet, heat 1 tablespoon of oil over medium-high heat. Cook the tofu for 3 to 4 minutes, then flip and cook for 2 to 3 minutes until browned. Add 1 tablespoon of tamari and half of the ginger. Stir and continue to cook until the tofu takes on the color of the tamari, about 2 more minutes. Remove from the skillet and set aside.

4. In a large bowl, toss the rice, carrot, remaining 1 tablespoon of tamari, and remaining ginger and mix well. Top with the tofu and scallion greens and serve with tamari on the side for drizzling, if desired.

Variation Tip: Add 1 cup of frozen edamame to the skillet along with the tamari and ginger to add even more vegetable content and protein.

PER SERVING: Calories: 335; Total Fat: 13g; Sodium: 534mg; Sugars: 2g; Carbohydrates: 43g; Fiber: 4g; Protein: 14g

Roasted Veggie and Buckwheat Tahini Bowl

Eggplant and zucchini are a perfect pair in this warm salad bowl. Look for buckwheat in natural food stores or order it online.

SERVES 4 / PREP TIME: 10 MINUTES, PLUS OVERNIGHT TO SOAK / COOK TIME: 15 MINUTES

8 ounces extra-firm tofu

1 large
 eggplant, chopped

2 small zucchinis, cut
 lengthwise then sliced

Olive oil, coconut
 oil, or avocado oil
 cooking spray

2 cups water

1 cup buckwheat groats,
 soaked in water
 overnight and drained

2 tablespoons tahini

2 tablespoons
 extra-virgin olive oil

Salt

Black pepper

1. Preheat the oven to 375°F.

2. Using several paper towels, press down on the tofu firmly to expel as much water as possible. Remove the paper towels and chop the tofu.

3. On a large baking sheet, toss the eggplant, zucchini, and tofu. Spray with cooking spray, toss the vegetables, then spray again.

4. Cook for 15 minutes, toss, and cook for 10 more minutes until browned.

5. In a small saucepot, bring the water and buckwheat to a boil. Reduce the heat and simmer for 12 to 15 minutes until just tender. Drain and transfer to a bowl.

6. While the vegetables and buckwheat are cooking, combine the tahini and oil in a small bowl. Season with salt and pepper.

7. To serve, divide the buckwheat among bowls and top with the roasted vegetables and tofu. Drizzle with the tahini dressing and serve.

Variation Tip: Add a handful of chopped romaine lettuce for extra texture.

PER SERVING: Calories: 353; Total Fat: 16g; Sodium: 63mg; Sugars: 8g; Carbohydrates: 44g; Fiber: 10g; Protein: 15g

FISH OR POULTRY ENTREES

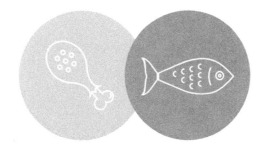

Avocado Tuna Salad Wraps

In this tuna salad, creamy, fatty avocado is used in place of mayonnaise. It is served with lettuce leaves here, but if you prefer a more substantial sandwich, place the lettuce and tuna inside two pieces of gluten-free bread.

SERVES 4 / PREP TIME: 10 MINUTES

3 (5-ounce) cans
  water-packed
  tuna, drained
1 English
  cucumber, chopped
2 avocados, chopped
¼ cup chopped fresh
  cilantro
Salt
Freshly ground
  black pepper
8 large lettuce leaves

1. In a small bowl, toss the tuna, cucumber, avocados, and cilantro. Season with salt and pepper.
2. Divide the salad among the lettuce leaves. Roll the leaves up and serve.

Variation Tip: Add your favorite seasoning to the tuna salad to personalize it to your taste. Add 1 small chopped dill pickle or substitute your favorite herbs, like basil, dill, or parsley, in place of the cilantro.

PER SERVING: Calories: 307; Total Fat: 18g; Sodium: 367mg; Sugars: 6g; Carbohydrates: 16g; Fiber: 9g; Protein: 24g

Sheet Pan Salmon, Asparagus, and Butternut Squash

Asparagus is rich in vitamin K and folic acid. It is also especially great in a sheet pan meal because it cooks so quickly. Using a simple seasoning, this filling meal is nearly all hands-off and tastes great year-round.

SERVES 4 / PREP TIME: 10 MINUTES / COOK TIME: 25 MINUTES

1 (16-ounce) bag butternut squash
2 tablespoons extra-virgin olive oil, divided
1 teaspoon dried thyme, divided
1 (1-pound) salmon fillet
1 pound asparagus, trimmed

1. Preheat the oven to 425°F.

2. On a large baking sheet, toss the butternut squash with 1 tablespoon of oil and ½ teaspoon of thyme. Bake for 10 minutes, remove from the oven, and stir. Clear a place in the center of the baking sheet.

3. Place the salmon in the center of the baking sheet. Arrange the asparagus around the salmon and cook for 15 minutes, until the salmon flakes easily with a fork and the squash and asparagus are tender.

Variation Tip: Look for frozen sweet potatoes and Brussels sprouts at the store to substitute for the butternut squash and asparagus.

PER SERVING: Calories: 295; Total Fat: 14g; Sodium: 57mg; Sugars: 5g; Carbohydrates: 18g; Fiber: 5g; Protein: 26g

Chicken Zucchini Noodle Soup

This comforting chicken noodle soup slow cooks for hours without needing your attention. If you use frozen vegetables, add them at the end along with the zucchini. Fresh vegetables should go in at the beginning, along with the chicken.

SERVES 4 / PREP TIME: 10 MINUTES / COOK TIME: 6 TO 8 HOURS

8 cups water

2 bone-in chicken breasts

1 cup chopped carrots

1 tablespoon Italian seasoning

1 tablespoon Onion- and Garlic-Infused Oil (page 110) or extra-virgin olive oil

1 teaspoon salt

½ teaspoon black pepper

1 (12-ounce) bag frozen spiralized zucchini

1 bunch scallions, green parts only, chopped

1. In a slow cooker, combine the water, chicken breasts, carrots, Italian seasoning, oil, salt, and pepper. Cover and cook for 6 to 8 hours on low.

2. Remove the chicken and set aside to cool. Add the zucchini and let cook for 3 to 5 minutes until tender.

3. When the chicken is cool enough to handle, shred the meat with two forks, then return to the slow cooker.

4. Spoon the soup into bowls and top with scallion greens to serve.

Variation Tip: To make the soup a bit heartier, add your favorite cooked gluten-free noodle instead of zucchini. Corn noodles are a good choice, but there are many other gluten-free options, such as rice- and lentil-based noodles, that would work great in this soup.

PER SERVING: Calories: 309; Total Fat: 17g; Sodium: 702mg; Sugars: 4g; Carbohydrates: 6g; Fiber: 2g; Protein: 32g

One-Pot Chicken, Beans, and Greens

One-pot meals streamline both cooking and cleanup. Chicken thighs are used for this dish, as they are juicy and tender. You are welcome to use chicken breasts in their place for a lower-fat option; just cut the breasts into thin strips and lightly brown them before adding the rice.

SERVES 4 / PREP TIME: 10 MINUTES / COOK TIME: 45 MINUTES

1 tablespoon Onion- and Garlic-Infused Oil (page 110) or extra-virgin olive oil
1 pound boneless, skinless chicken thighs
1 cup brown rice
Salt
Black pepper
1¾ cups water
1 bunch collard greens, stemmed and chopped
1 (15-ounce) can cannellini beans, drained and rinsed

1. In a medium pot, heat the oil over medium heat. Add the chicken and brown on both sides, flipping once, for about 10 minutes.

2. Add the rice, salt, and pepper and stir to combine. Pour in the water. Place the collards and beans on top without stirring, cover, and reduce the heat to low. Cook for 30 to 35 minutes, until the rice absorbs all the water. Let stand for 10 minutes. Stir to combine, season with salt and pepper, and serve.

Variation Tip: Make this vegetarian by omitting the chicken and using 8 ounces of chopped, pressed firm tofu. Fry the tofu in step 1, until browned, then continue with the recipe as written.

PER SERVING: Calories: 424; Total Fat: 7g; Sodium: 107mg; Sugars: 1g; Carbohydrates: 54g; Fiber: 8g; Protein: 36g

Slow Cooker White Chicken Chili

It's hard to get that chili flavor without the classic nightshades that typically go into it, but this white chicken chili is super easy and gives you that great chili taste without the tomatoes and chilis. This chili also takes very little effort.

SERVES 6 / PREP TIME: 10 MINUTES / COOK TIME: 6 TO 8 HOURS

1 pound boneless, skinless chicken thighs

2 (15-ounce) cans cannellini beans, drained and rinsed

6 cups water

1 teaspoon ground cumin

Salt

Black pepper

1 avocado, sliced

¼ cup chopped fresh cilantro

Juice of 1 lime

1. In a slow cooker, combine the chicken, beans, water, cumin, salt, and pepper. Cover and cook on low for 6 to 8 hours.

2. Taste and season with more salt and pepper as needed. Serve in bowls, topped with avocado, cilantro, and lime juice.

Variation Tip: Top each bowl of soup with a tablespoon of dairy-free cheese, if desired.

PER SERVING: Calories: 265; Total Fat: 8g; Sodium: 103mg; Sugars: 1g; Carbohydrates: 25g; Fiber: 11g; Protein: 24g

BONUS RECIPES

Onion- and Garlic-Infused Oil

This is a great substitute for using onion and garlic in recipes, especially for people with irritable bowel syndrome, who may experience increased discomfort after eating these high FODMAP foods.

MAKES ½ CUP / PREP TIME: 5 MINUTES / COOK TIME: 5 MINUTES, PLUS 1 HOUR RESTING TIME

½ cup extra-virgin olive oil

1 onion, quartered

3 garlic cloves, crushed

1. In a small pot, slowly heat the oil, onion, and garlic over low heat until the garlic and onion have tiny bubbles rising from them and the oil is hot. Remove from the heat and let cool for about 1 hour, until at room temperature.

2. Using a strainer, remove the onion and garlic pieces from the oil and discard. Transfer the cooled oil to an airtight container and refrigerate for up to 3 or 4 days.

PER SERVING (1 TABLESPOON): Calories: 84; Total Fat: 9g; Sodium: 1mg; Sugars: 0g; Carbohydrates: 1g; Fiber: 0g; Protein: 0g

Golden Milk

This recipe is a great anti-inflammatory and immune-boosting drink for days when your pain levels are peaking. Adding black pepper increases the bio-availability of turmeric, which means your body can access its pain-relieving properties more easily.

MAKES 1 CUP / PREP TIME: 2 MINUTES / COOK TIME: 3 TO 4 MINUTES

1 cup non-dairy milk
½ teaspoon turmeric
1 tablespoon honey or maple syrup
Dash black pepper
⅛ teaspoon of ginger (optional)
¼ teaspoon cinnamon (optional)

Mix the ingredients in a saucepan. Warm at medium heat for about 3 minutes. Serve and enjoy!

PER SERVING (1 SERVING): Calories: 188; Total Fat: 4g; Sodium: 127mg; Sugars: 22g; Carbohydrates: 30g; Fiber: 2g; Protein: 8g

CHAPTER 5
FOUR WEEKS TO IMPROVE PHYSICAL MOVEMENT

You have made it to our third and final monthly plan together. The goal for this month is to increase flexibility and decrease pain with movement. As always, how you incorporate this month's plan is up to you. You can continue to rest, relax, and eat an anti-inflammatory diet while incorporating movement, or you can focus just on increasing movement this month if that is easier for you. Although this book provides a layout for 28-day plans, you can continue trying out the different suggestions in this book until you find the combination that works best for you.

THE TANGLE OF FASCIA, INFLAMMATION, AND PAIN

You may have heard the term "fascia" and wondered exactly what it is and how it relates to the pain and stiffness that you are experiencing. Fascia is a band of connective tissue made up mostly of collagen. It is present throughout our bodies, and it allows different parts of our bodies to work as an integrated whole. Fascia looks similar to a spider's web but is very dense and surrounds every bone, nerve, blood vessel, organ, and muscle, and helps hold them in place. All of the roles of fascia in the body are still being studied. Until the last decade or so, researchers tended to overlook fascia, focusing on other elements of human anatomy like muscle and bone. (You won't see fascia represented on those diagrams of the musculoskeletal system at your doctor's office!)

Fascia is integral to the way we move, and it keeps our bodies flexible yet structured. These tissues are able to tense or relax independent of the muscles they surround, which means they can prevent overstretching. When fascia is irritated or damaged, it thickens and hardens as a means to protect the underlying structure. This causes it to lose its flexibility and makes movement much more difficult and painful.

Fascia is also deeply connected to our nervous system. Fascia can tighten in response to injury or negative emotions, making movement much more difficult. Pain associated with irritated fascia can be felt throughout the body, and not necessarily just the location that suffered the initial trauma. A lack of stretching, dehydration, or physical and emotional trauma can all cause irritation to the fascia. Fortunately, none of this has to be permanent. *The British Journal of Sports Medicine* published a review of research on fascial tissue in 2018, confirming that exercise and stretching can, in fact, reduce the pain and inflammation caused by damaged fascia. This is great news for those with fibromyalgia. You have already been improving your rest, emotions, and diet to decrease inflammation. Now, with the right type of movement, you can also soothe your internal tissues and reduce generalized pain.

WHY THERAPEUTIC MOVEMENT?

Low-impact therapeutic movement is beneficial for people with fibromyalgia. Therapeutic movement is used to help people recover from physical or emotional illness, or from disability. Here is a list of some of the most popular forms of therapeutic movement that can improve quality of life for people with this chronic pain syndrome, many of which can be done at home (look for YouTube tutorials if you're unsure where to start):

- **Biking** is easy on the joints and can help reduce stress and improve balance and flexibility. If you're biking around your neighborhood, you can go at your own gentle pace; depending on where you live, you can also combine biking with errands (if you have the energy). A stationary bike can be used at home and is often incorporated into physical therapy routines as well.
- **Dance** is a great form of therapeutic movement. It is fun and helps alleviate stress. It has physical, emotional, and cognitive benefits. Dance therapy may be covered by some private insurance plans.
- **Pilates** is a form of exercise that focuses on strengthening the core and increasing flexibility. It has been incorporated into many physical therapy routines, and it can be covered by medical insurance as a form of physical therapy. There are also Pilates routines that can be done at home with little or no equipment.
- **Qigong** originated in China and is a mind and body practice. It involves gentle movement, breathing, self-massage, and meditative focus to open the flow of energy in the meridians used in Chinese medicine. Qigong can also be done at home.
- **Swimming** and water exercise are very low-impact forms of movement. The water takes the stress off the joints, which makes it easier to move without pain. Swimming can improve flexibility, circulation, strength, and lung capacity. If you have difficulty doing water aerobics or strengthening exercises due to joint pain, doing them in a warm water pool may work better for you. Water exercise can sometimes

be incorporated into physical therapy, and thus can be covered by insurance.

- **Tai chi** originated in China as a martial art. It involves very slow and gentle movements. In tai chi, unlike yoga, the muscles are always relaxed and never tensed. It can improve strength, balance, and flexibility and decrease anxiety and stress. If you are on Medicare, look into what exercise benefits might be covered.

- **Walking** supports physical and emotional health. It increases circulation and oxygenation throughout the body, and its rhythmic pacing is very soothing and can lower stress hormones.

- **Yoga** originated in India as a spiritual practice. Over the course of its long history, yoga has become popular worldwide as a form of body movement to promote physical and emotional health. There are many different studios and gyms offering yoga classes, but it can also be done at your own pace in the comfort of your own home.

STRATEGIES FOR INCREASING PHYSICAL MOVEMENT

Increasing physical movement does not have to involve a formal exercise routine. Any gentle movement will be beneficial, as it will warm up muscles that are far too often achy and stiff. Here are a few simple ways that you can increase physical movement by working it into your daily routine:

Stretch before getting out of bed. Most of the stretches and exercises at the end of this chapter can be done in the comfort of your own bed. Stretching first thing in the morning is actually a great way to decrease pain and stiffness and be more functional throughout the day.

Catch up on household chores. Even doing some cleaning at home can be a great way to increase movement. If your energy levels permit, you can mop and sweep floors and wash, dry, and put away dishes. These are all forms of movement and, thus, forms of exercise. Of course, something taxing like scrubbing floors may not be a good chore to do, since it can be tiring and leave you achy.

Walking. Just increasing the amount of walking you do is something to celebrate. You can walk around your house, walk to a nearby park, or walk around your favorite store. Whatever your energy levels permit is fine. Even if you can only walk for three minutes at first, you've done something positive for yourself. You can try another three minutes later on in the day or the next day.

Gardening. If you like gardening, this can be a great way to get you outdoors and moving around. Whether you are planting new seeds, moving plants from pots to the ground, or just going outside to water and check on your plants, these will all increase physical movement. You also benefit from sunshine, which decreases inflammation and triggers vitamin D production in the body.

With fibromyalgia, there can be days when you are in too much pain to move. This is a good time to focus instead on relaxing and getting as much pain relief as possible. Warming your body will help decrease the inflammation and increase relaxation. The warm aromatherapy bath listed under the Remedies for Relaxation section (page 41) would be great for a day like this. If you have heating pads or blankets that you can place over the most painful areas, those can help as well. You can also try a short sunbath if the weather permits. Sitting outdoors and practicing your deep breathing under the sun will have a relaxing and anti-inflammatory effect and can also increase energy. Try one of the pain-relieving supplements mentioned in chapter 2, like Full Life Reuma-Art, if they are not contraindicated with any medications you may be taking. You can also warm the body with foods. Try recipes from chapter 4 with warming spices like turmeric, ginger, cinnamon, and cumin. Drinking turmeric can provide relief much faster than taking a turmeric supplement. Try the recipe for Golden Milk that appears on page 111. If you find relief from any of these suggestions, you may find yourself able to at least do some of the stretches and move a little bit around your home.

BEST PRACTICES FOR SAFE, INJURY-FREE PROGRESS

Your exercise routine, like everything else discussed in this book, will be customized by you, for you, based on your needs and tolerance level. Also keep in mind that your tolerance levels may vary from day to day. Don't feel pressured to accomplish a certain amount or type of exercise one day, even if you were able to do it successfully a few days ago. Remember that even on days you feel well, it is best that you take things slowly and not push yourself too much, because this can cause a flare-up. Here are several tips to assist you in increasing physical movement safely:

- The key is to exercise slowly and gently. It may be necessary to modify certain exercises if they are too complicated for you to do them without increasing your pain or aggravating a preexisting injury.
- Break your exercise routine apart into different sessions. If your goal is 15 minutes of exercise each day, split your routine into sessions of five or 10 minutes. You can make a goal that's even smaller: One minute of exercise. If you feel all right after one minute, you can do more, or not. Either way, you have moved a little bit and you have met your goal. The point is to be kind to yourself. Setting small goals can be the path to success.
- Exercise at the time of day you normally feel the least amount of pain and/or the time you feel the most energetic.
- Stick to low-impact exercises like the ones mentioned in this chapter. High-intensity or high-impact exercises have a greater risk for injury or causing a flare-up.
- Try to stretch daily. Stretches should not be painful. If you are stretching to the point that it causes pain, you may have gone too deep into the stretch. Be gentle with yourself.
- Proper breathing will ensure muscle relaxation and oxygenation. When beginning an exercise, you first inhale and then exhale slowly as you perform the movement causing the most muscle exertion.

- Allow enough time for recovery between exercises. After strength training, you will likely need at least 48 hours to recover, depending on the severity of your symptoms. Remember that rest is necessary for proper healing, and when you exercise, you need to rest and heal afterward.
- Keep track of exercises you are doing, as well as your pain and fatigue levels the days after. This will help you determine how much exercise your body can tolerate. Over time, the exercise should decrease pain and increase energy. If exercising has caused a flare-up, you may have done too much.

YOUR GENTLE 28-DAY MOVEMENT PLAN

Assess your current physical state. You may be feeling some pain and/or stiffness, and movement can seem daunting when we're already in pain. However, creating a routine for regular physical movement will actually decrease your pain and increase your flexibility over time. You definitely do not need to wait until you are pain-free to start moving, but you can use your pain levels to help you determine how much physical activity you can do. On days where pain levels are higher, try walking for just one minute, or doing some stretches in bed. If even that is too much, you can instead focus on some of the relaxation remedies from chapter 3 and work on incorporating movement the following day. Remember to move gently. You want to do these exercises slowly and modify them whenever necessary so that you are able to complete the exercise without increasing the amount of pain you are in. Do not overdo it.

Think about what time in your day you can set aside for movement. How much movement do you think you can incorporate safely? In order to fill out the worksheet for this month's plan, you will need to:

- Commit to movement one to three times per day. If you are in severe pain, you can commit to movement every other day.
- Choose three stretches or exercises from the 20 Stretches and Exercises section (page 124) to do daily for the next seven days. You can choose different ones each week.
- Remember to complete the Tracking Symptoms, Treatments, and Results worksheet found on pages 28 and 29 at the end of each day to monitor your progress.

Write the name of the stretch or exercise you want to try in the blank spaces.
Cross out each day that you successfully complete it to log your progress.

Stretch or Exercise #1						
Week 1						
Mon	Tues	Wed	Thur	Fri	Sat	Sun
Week 2						
Mon	Tues	Wed	Thur	Fri	Sat	Sun
Week 3						
Mon	Tues	Wed	Thur	Fri	Sat	Sun
Week 4						
Mon	Tues	Wed	Thur	Fri	Sat	Sun

Stretch or Exercise #2						
Week 1						
Mon	Tues	Wed	Thur	Fri	Sat	Sun
Week 2						
Mon	Tues	Wed	Thur	Fri	Sat	Sun
Week 3						
Mon	Tues	Wed	Thur	Fri	Sat	Sun
Week 4						
Mon	Tues	Wed	Thur	Fri	Sat	Sun

Stretch or Exercise #3						
Week 1						
Mon	Tues	Wed	Thur	Fri	Sat	Sun
Week 2						
Mon	Tues	Wed	Thur	Fri	Sat	Sun
Week 3						
Mon	Tues	Wed	Thur	Fri	Sat	Sun
Week 4						
Mon	Tues	Wed	Thur	Fri	Sat	Sun

NECK STRETCH

Stretching your neck can increase flexibility and decrease pain in that area. This is a great stretch to do first thing in the morning or during the day if you feel tension or tightness building.

Instructions

1. Hold your hands together behind your back while standing or sitting.

2. Take a deep breath. As you exhale, move your head to look up toward the ceiling.

3. As you inhale, move your head back to a neutral position looking straight ahead.

4. Repeat steps 2 and 3 for a total of seven repetitions.

5. Take a deep breath. As you exhale, move your head down to bring your chin toward your chest.

6. Inhale again, bringing your head back to a neutral position looking straight ahead.

7. Repeat steps 5 and 6 for a total of seven repetitions.

8. Take a deep breath. As you exhale, gently pull your neck to the right.

9. Take another deep breath. As you exhale, gently pull your neck to the left.

10. Repeat steps 8 and 9 for a total of seven repetitions.

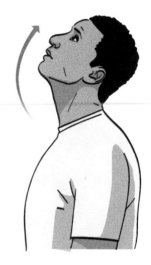

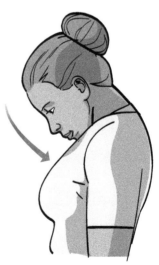

Tip: As you pull your neck from side to side, you only need to pull enough to feel the stretch and never to the point that it becomes painful. Use the repetitions as a goal. If you cannot do all seven, do as many as you can and increase the repetitions over time as your flexibility improves. Track your progress in your symptoms log.

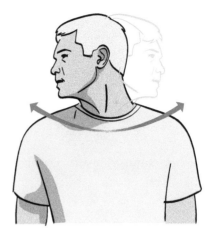

SHOULDER ROLLS

This is a very simple way to reduce tightness in the shoulders. Try this stretch before any upper body exercises. You should also try this before doing any chores requiring you to hold, carry, or reach for things over your head.

Instructions

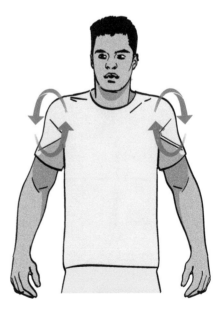

1. Stand or sit with your arms at your sides and your back straight.

2. Slowly lift both of your shoulders up toward your ears, and then back, as if squeezing your shoulder blades together.

3. Then relax and return your shoulders back to their neutral position.

4. Continue this for a total of seven repetitions.

CHEST STRETCH

A tight chest pulls shoulders forward and causes poor posture. By keeping the chest muscles loose and flexible, you can improve your posture and reduce pain and tension in the upper back and shoulders.

Instructions

1. While standing or sitting upright, take a deep breath and place both hands over your ears, with your elbows pointing to the front.

2. As you exhale, open your arms wide so that the elbows are now pointing to the sides.

3. Hold this stretch for three to five seconds and then repeat the stretch seven times.

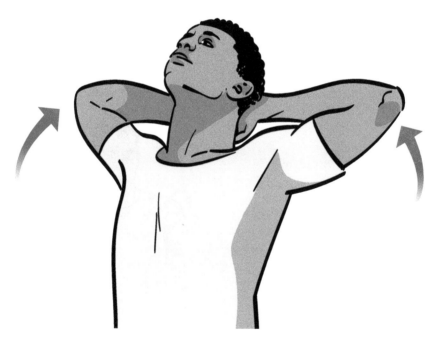

CAT-COW STRETCH

This stretch can be great for improving posture and balance. Stretching out your spine improves circulation along the spine and also has a calming effect on the body. This is especially good for when you have been sitting for extended periods of time or have had a stressful day.

Instructions

1. Get on your hands and knees on the floor.

2. Position your hands under your shoulders and your knees under your hips.

3. Start with your spine parallel to the floor.

4. Inhale and arch your back by tilting your pelvis so that your tailbone sticks up. Your head should be facing forward.

5. Exhale and round out your spine so that your tailbone is tucked in, your spine is round, and your head is facing your belly.

6. Repeat this for a total of seven breaths.

7. Return to a position where your spine is parallel to the floor before you get up.

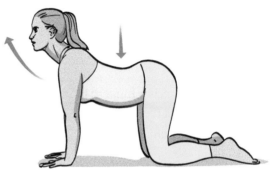

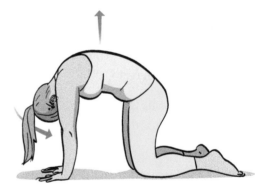

Tip: If getting on your hands and knees is too difficult or painful on the joints, this same exercise can be done while sitting in a chair or in bed. A neutral spine would be parallel to the walls in your house. You can still arch your spine while inhaling and round your spine while exhaling.

WRIST STRETCH

This stretch reduces risk of injury and increases flexibility in the wrist. If you find your hands are very stiff as you perform your daily tasks, starting and ending your day with wrist stretches could help you.

Instructions

1. Extend your arm in front of you with your palm facing down.

2. Bend your wrist so that your hand is pointing up.

3. Use your other hand to bend your wrist farther until you feel a good stretch.

4. Hold the stretch for about 10 seconds.

5. Release your hand and move it back to a neutral position with your palm facing up.

6. Bend your wrist so that your hand is pointing down.

7. Use your other hand to bend your wrist farther until you feel a good stretch.

8. Hold the stretch for about 10 seconds.

9. Repeat two or three times, and then do the same with the other arm.

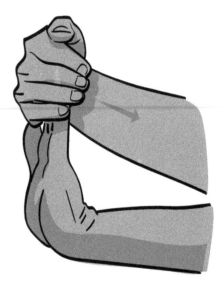

Tip: Remember that stretching should not be painful. Do not stretch to the point that it causes pain.

KNEE TO CHEST

This stretch is effective for releasing tension in the lower spine. It can be done in bed first thing in the morning. You can also try it at the end of the day, when tension in your body has built up.

Instructions

1. Lie on your back and bend your knees.

2. Use your hands to gently pull one knee toward your chest.

3. Hold for about five seconds, then lower your leg.

4. Repeat the exercise with the other leg.

5. Alternate between legs for a total of seven repetitions on each leg.

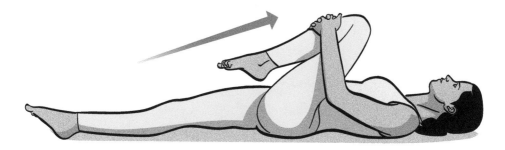

Tip: For a deeper stretch, you can leave your legs extended instead of beginning with your knees bent.

ANKLE CIRCLES

Ankle circles improve the range of motion. If you are feeling ankle pain or stiffness, you can try this stretch. If you have any injury in your ankle, make sure to ask your healthcare provider whether this type of movement is safe.

Instructions

1. While sitting or lying down, move one of your ankles as if you were tracing a circle with your toe. Repeat this for a total of seven circles clockwise, then seven circles counterclockwise.

2. Relax that ankle and repeat the exercise with the other foot.

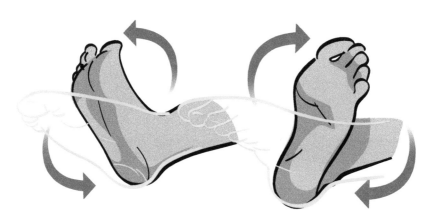

HEEL SLIDES

This exercise can increase the range of motion in the knee while stretching and strengthening the muscles and ligaments around the leg.

Instructions

1. Lie on your back with your legs extended.

2. Bending one knee, slowly and gently slide the heel of your foot straight back toward your buttocks as far as you can.

3. Then slowly extend your leg.

4. Gently repeat with the other foot. Continue alternating legs for a total of seven repetitions on each leg.

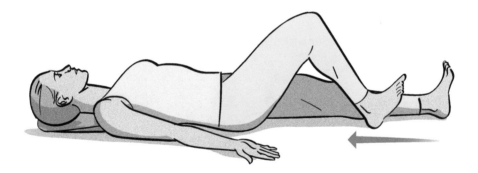

SPINAL TWIST

This stretch will help release tension in the low back area. This area is very prone to injury from lifting and bending with improper form. Strengthening the abdomen and back and stretching these muscles can prevent injury and decrease discomfort.

Instructions

1. Lie on your back with your knees bent.

2. Gently pull both legs to one side as far as you can without moving your torso.

3. Hold for about three seconds.

4. Gently pull both legs to the opposite side as far as you can without moving your torso.

5. Hold for about three seconds.

6. Continue to alternate for a total of seven repetitions on each side.

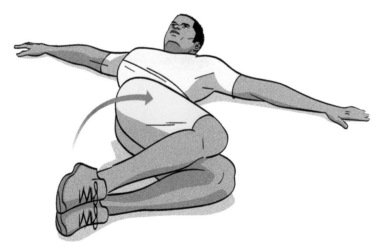

Tip: A twisting motion is bad for different types of back injuries. If you have a back injury, ask your healthcare provider before trying this stretch.

CHILD'S POSE

This pose reduces stress and fatigue. It stretches the hips, thighs, and ankles. This is a nice stretch to do at the end of an exercise routine, at the end of the day, or while meditating.

Instructions

1. Begin on your hands and knees.

2. Spread your knees apart while keeping your big toes touching.

3. Sit back until your buttocks are resting on your feet as you take a deep breath.

4. As you exhale, lean forward and bring your torso toward your thighs as you extend your arms, palms facing down.

5. Continue to take deep breaths and lengthen your arms while relaxing the rest of your body.

6. Hold this position for at least five deep breaths. You can hold this pose for as long as you feel comfortable.

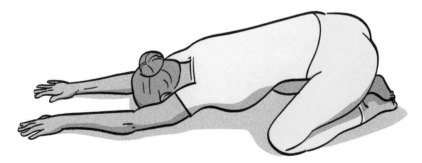

Tip: Avoid this pose if you have any knee injuries. If you are unable to rest your buttocks on your feet, you can place a pillow between your thighs and calves. You can also add padding under your feet and face for comfort. If extending your arms makes it difficult to relax, you can also rest your arms by your thighs.

SHOULDER PRESS

This exercise is a very gentle way of strengthening the back and shoulders. It is beneficial for anyone who carries a lot of tension in this area, has poor posture, or is experiencing shoulder and back pain.

Instructions

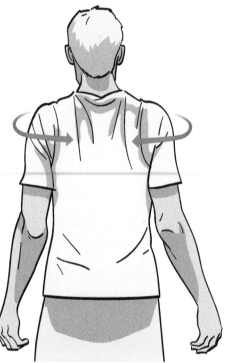

1. Push your shoulders back as if trying to squeeze your shoulder blades together.

2. Raise your shoulders up toward your ears and then back down.

3. Repeat for three sets of seven repetitions.

4. Between sets, you can relax your shoulders by bringing them back to neutral.

Tip: Try not to strain your neck as you lift and push your shoulders back. If you notice yourself holding tension in other parts of your body, relax them and try again.

SCAPULAR WALL REPS

This exercise will help strengthen your upper back, which is necessary to maintain proper posture and prevent injury.

Instructions

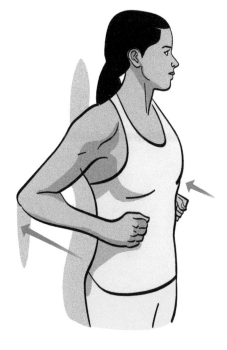

1. Stand with your back against a wall and your feet about shoulder-width apart.

2. As you inhale, bend your arms with your elbows touching the wall.

3. As you exhale, press your elbows against the wall and drive your body off the wall with your chest pushed forward, squeezing your buttocks and your shoulder blades down and back.

4. Relax your back against the wall again.

5. Repeat for three sets of seven repetitions.

Tip: Make sure you are not shrugging your shoulders or arching your back. Your core should be moving forward in a straight line as your elbows press against the wall. Try to keep your neck relaxed. The tension should be felt in your back.

CHEST PRESS

This exercise is helpful for anyone suffering from chronic pain or fatigue, because it requires almost no movement. You simply isolate, tense, and hold the muscle group you are seeking to strengthen.

Instructions

1. Clasp your hands together in front of your chest.

2. Keep your shoulders back and tense your chest muscles as you push them forward.

3. Hold this for about 10 seconds.

4. Repeat three to five times.

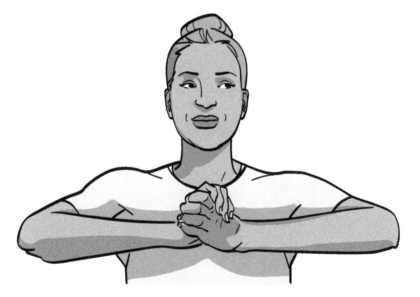

Tip: Keep the neck, hands, and wrists relaxed. Focus on isolating and tensing the chest muscles during the exercise. If you feel the tension building somewhere else, stop and try again.

THIGH SLIDES

This exercise is a modified, easier form of crunches that can strengthen your abdominal muscles. A strong core is necessary for good posture and preventing back injuries. A strong core can also help ease pain from existing back injuries.

Instructions

1. Lie on your back with your knees bent.

2. Place your hands on your thighs and take a deep breath.

3. As you exhale, pull your navel up and gently slide your hands up toward your knees, keeping your back as straight as possible.

4. As you inhale, bring your hands back down your thighs.

5. Repeat for a total of seven thigh slides.

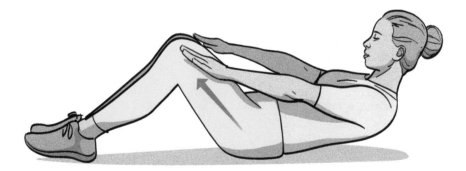

Tip: Be careful not to strain your neck. Sometimes touching the roof of your mouth with your tongue can help prevent you from straining your neck.

LEG EXTENSIONS

This exercise will strengthen the muscle group on the front of your thigh. We use these muscles—quadriceps—to sit, stand, squat, and lunge. These seated leg extensions allow you to start working these muscles without requiring the balance needed to perform different squats and lunges.

Instructions

1. Sit in a chair with your back straight and your feet on the floor.

2. As you exhale, keep your back straight, tense your abdominal muscles, and elevate your right leg until it is parallel to the floor.

3. Keep the leg elevated for about 15 seconds. Continue taking deep breaths.

4. Relax the leg back down with both feet on the floor.

5. Repeat with the left leg.

6. Do this three to five times on each leg.

Tip: Try not to lean to the sides as you elevate your legs. If you need to, you can hold the sides of your chair for balance. Elevate only as far as you can without losing form. If you are unable to keep your legs elevated for 15 seconds, don't force it. Keep them elevated as long as you can without shaking or pain.

SQUATS

Every time we sit, stand, get in and out of a car, or even go down stairs, we're doing a type of squat. Practicing squats with proper form can help strengthen the legs and buttocks and make these common movements easier and less painful.

Instructions

1. Stand with your feet shoulder-width apart, pointing slightly outward.

2. Look straight ahead, with your shoulders back. Tighten your abs.

3. Take a deep breath. As you exhale, bend your knees while moving your buttocks backward, as if you were taking a seat. Keep your upper body straight, facing forward as you squat down.

4. As you inhale again, lift yourself back to a standing position.

5. Repeat this one to three times per set. Try to do seven to ten sets, taking breaks in between.

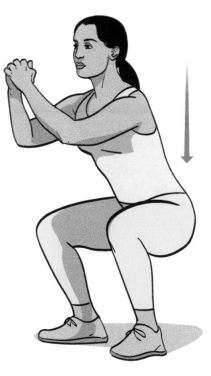

Tip: If a standing squat feels too difficult, you can modify this exercise by doing the squats up against a wall. Keep your back straight against the wall and squat down during exhales and come back up when inhaling.

BRIDGES

This exercise strengthens the lower body muscles while relaxing the upper body muscles. It can help calm the body and alleviate stress.

Instructions

1. Place a mat or thick towel on the floor. Lie down on your back.

2. Bend your knees so that both feet are flat on the floor.

3. Straighten your arms by your sides and take a deep breath.

4. As you exhale, lift your tailbone off the floor as high as you can while squeezing your buttocks.

5. Hold this pose for five to ten seconds while continuing to take deep breaths.

6. Exhale as you slowly lower your back toward the floor.

7. Each set is one to three bridges. Try to do seven sets, resting in between sets.

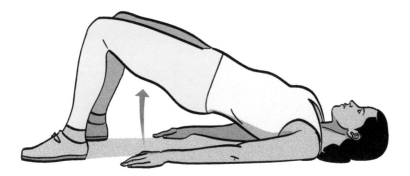

Tip: Placing a rolled towel or blanket under your shoulders can make this position more comfortable. If you have a neck injury, avoid this exercise. If you are unable to do seven repetitions, do whatever you can and write down how much you were able to do on your worksheet.

SIMPLE LEG EXERCISES

Strengthening the muscles in the inner and outer hips improves stability in the legs. We use these muscles to open and close our legs and to maintain balance. These two exercises are very simple and can be done in your bed.

Instructions

1. Lie on your side with a pillow under your head, with your legs extended and your feet together.

2. Raise your top leg as high as you can without rotating your pelvis.

3. Gently lower the leg back down.

4. Repeat this for a total of seven to ten repetitions.

5. Flip over to your other side and do the same with the opposite leg.

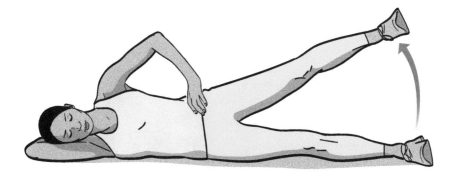

Modified: If raising your entire leg is too complicated, you can lie on your side with your knees bent. Keep your heels together, aligned with your shoulders. Then, raise the top leg without rotating your hip or separating your heels.

Tip: This movement should be very slow and gentle. Raising the top leg just three or four inches is enough for this exercise.

Instructions

1. Lie flat on your back.

2. Bend your knees and keep your feet flat on the floor or bed.

3. Place a pillow, folded bed sheet, or ball between your thighs, just above the knee.

4. Take a deep breath and, as you exhale, press the pillow, sheet, or ball with your inner thighs.

5. Relax your legs as you inhale.

6. Repeat this for a total of seven compressions.

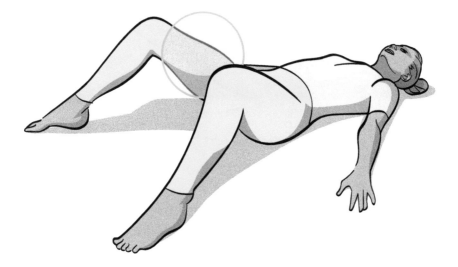

HEEL RAISES

This exercise strengthens the calf muscles and can be beneficial for people with calf pain or lower leg injuries. It works on the knees, ankles, feet, and calves. If no injury is present, strengthening the calves can help prevent injury in the future. (Please be sure to check with your doctor before starting this exercise if you have an injury, though.)

Instructions

1. Stand up straight, using a counter or chair for balance in front of you.

2. Rise up so that you are standing on your toes.

3. Hold this for three to five seconds, then lower yourself back onto your heels.

4. Repeat seven times. Try to do seven repetitions three times.

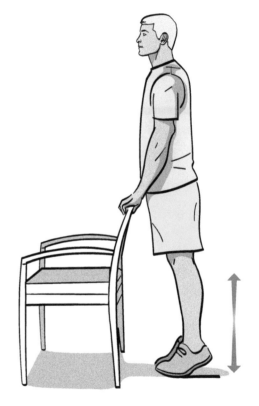

FINAL THOUGHT

Congratulations! You have made it through three months of trying out new ways to address the most vital foundations of health. I hope you are proud of yourself for having the courage and determination to make it this far. You may be wondering what's next. You are equipped with a better understanding of what a holistic healing approach looks like, and you have also learned a little bit more about what practices worked or didn't work for you. There are at least a few options that you can consider moving forward.

If you noticed there was a specific area (emotional health, nutrition, or movement) where you felt the most progress, or where you had the most difficulty being consistent, you can go back and focus on that area from here on out.

If you felt too overwhelmed before to try addressing all three areas together, but feel more confident now that you have seen the results, you can revisit multiple areas as well.

If you have already gone back and followed the general recommendations from this book for quite some time and seen progress, it may be time to invest in a holistic consultation with a practitioner who can create an individualized plan for you.

Most important, hold on to what was good, valuable, or beneficial. Continue to incorporate what you have learned into your lifestyle and, if possible, share it with others. Applying your knowledge gives you the power to change your current situation for the better. Sharing the knowledge gives you the power of influencing that change in others.

RESOURCES

ORGANIZATIONS

National Fibromyalgia & Chronic Pain Association
fibroandpain.org

Fibromyalgia Coalition International
fibrocoalition.org

American Fibromyalgia Syndrome Association, Inc.
afsafund.org

Hope Instilled: An Oasis from the Darkness of Pain
hopeinstilled.org

These organizations provide several resources to people with fibromyalgia ranging from up-to-date research on treatment options to support groups and beyond.

FIBROMYALGIA SUPPORT GROUPS BY STATE

fibroandpain.org/support-groups
This is a directory to locate fibromyalgia support groups around the country. You can select your state to see a list of the groups in your area and find additional information about them.

Labs
mymedlab.com
directlabs.com
mylabsforlife.com
walkinlab.com

These are different labs where you can order your own tests. In order to find out which underlying issues may be causing your fibromyalgia, it may require some testing. These tests are not always covered by insurance, and many medical doctors may not order them.

HERB/DRUG INTERACTION CHECKER

naturaldatabaseconsumer
.therapeuticresearch.com

This is a great tool for confirming any possible interaction between herbs, supplements, or drugs. Several of the herbs mentioned in this book can interact with the drugs most commonly prescribed for fibromyalgia and are therefore contraindicated. This is for informational purposes and should not replace checking with your doctor before making any changes to any medications you are taking.

WHERE TO BUY SUPPLEMENTS AND ESSENTIAL OILS

Your local health-food store should have plenty of supplements and essential oils to choose from. But if you don't have access to a health-food store, you can purchase the following brands online directly from the brands' sites. Additionally, there are always sites like Amazon, the Vitamin Shoppe, and iHerb.

Supplement Brands: NOW, New Chapter, Organixx, Gaia, Hallelujah Diet, Life Extension, Source Naturals, Solaray, Solgar, Nature's Way, Natural Calm (for magnesium specifically)

Essential Oil Brands: NOW, doTerra, Young Living, Organixx

Resource for Financial Difficulty
NeedHelpPayingBills.com

This site is a great resource for finding out what type of assistance is available to you. There is a menu on the left with options to direct your search. You can find a food pantry directory, information about getting free prescriptions, free medical care, help paying bills, and much more.

REFERENCES

Ali, Ather, and Paul L. McCarthy. "Complementary and Integrative Methods in Fibromyalgia." *Pediatrics in Review* 35, no. 12 (December 2014): 510–8. doi:10.1542/pir.35-12-510.

Amen, Daniel G. *Change Your Brain, Change Your Life.* 2nd ed., London: Piatus, 2016.

Bennett, Robert, and David Nelson. "Cognitive Behavioral Therapy for Fibromyalgia." *Nature Clinical Practice Rheumatology* 2, no. 8 (September 2006): 416–24. doi:10.1038/ncprheum0245.

Benson, Herbert, and Miriam Z. Klipper. *The Relaxation Response.* New York: Harper Collins, 2009.

Bjørklund, Geir, Maryam Dadar, Salvatore Chirumbolo, and Jan Aaseth. "Fibromyalgia and Nutrition: Therapeutic Possibilities?" *Biomedicine & Pharmacotherapy* 103 (July 2018): 531–8. doi:10.1016/j.biopha.2018.04.056.

Bordoni, Bruno, and Fabiola Marelli. "Emotions in Motion: Myofascial Interoception." *Complementary Medicine Research* 24, no. 2 (April 2017): 110–3. doi:10.1159/000464149.

Bordoni, Bruno, Kavin Sugumar, and Matthew Varacallo. "Myofascial Pain." *Stat*Pearls. Last modified March 15, 2020. StatPearls.com /kb/viewarticle/25475.

Breit, Sigrid, Aleksandra Kupferberg, Gerhard Rogler, and Gregor Hasler. "Vagus Nerve as Modulator of the Brain–Gut Axis in Psychiatric and Inflammatory Disorders." *Frontiers in Psychiatry* 13, no. 9 (March 2018): 44. doi:10.3389/ fpsyt.2018.00044.

Busch, Angela J., Sandra C. Webber, Mary Brachaniec, Julia Bidonde, Vanina Dal Bello-Haas, Adrienne D. Danyliw, Tom J. Overend, Rachel S. Richards, Anuradha Sawant, and Candice L. Schachter. "Exercise Therapy for Fibromyalgia." *Current Pain and Headache Reports* 15, no. 5 (October 2011): 358–67. doi:10.1007/s11916-011-0214-2.

Buskila, Dan, Lily Neumann, Genady Vaisberg, Daphna Alkalay, and Frederick Wolfe. "Increased Rates of Fibromyalgia Following Cervical Spine Injury. A Controlled Study of 161 Cases of Traumatic Injury." *Arthritis & Rheumatology* 40, no. 3 (March 1997): 446–52. doi: 10.1002 /art.1780400310.

Buyukkose, Mehves, Erkan Kozanoglu, Sibel Basaran, Ozlem Bayramoglu, and Fugen Yarkin. "Seroprevalence of Parvovirus B19 in Fibromyalgia Syndrome." *Clinical Rheumatology* 28, no. 3 (March 2009): 305–9. doi:10.1007 /s10067-008-1044-4.

Calder, Philip C. "Omega-3 Fatty Acids and Inflammatory Processes." *Nutrients* 2, no. 3 (March 2010): 355–74. doi:10.3390/nu2030355.

Castro-Sánchez, Adelaida María, Guillermo A. Matarán-Peñarrocha, José Granero-Molina, Gabriel Aguilera-Manrique, José Manuel Quesada-Rubio, and Carmen Moreno-Lorenzo. "Benefits of Massage-Myofascial Release Therapy on Pain, Anxiety, Quality of Sleep, Depression, and Quality of Life in Patients with Fibromyalgia." *Evidence-Based Complementary and Alternative Medicine* (December 2010). doi:10.1155/2011/561753.

Church, Dawson. *The Genie in Your Genes: Epigenetic Medicine and the New Biology of Intention.* New York: Energy Psychology Press, 2014.

Clauw, Daniel J., Lesley M. Arnold, and Bill H. McCarberg for the FibroCollaborative. "The Science of Fibromyalgia." *Mayo Clinic Proceedings* 86, no. 9 (September 2011): 907–11. doi:10.4065 /mcp.2011.0206.

D'Aoust, Rita F., Alicia Gill Rossiter, Amanda Elliott, Ming Ji, Cecile Lengacher, and Maureen Groer. "Women Veterans, a Population at Risk for Fibromyalgia: The Associations between Fibromyalgia, Symptoms, and Quality of Life." *Military Medicine* 182, no. 7 (July 2017): e1828–35. doi:10.7205 /MILMED-D-15-00557.

Dotan, Idit, Klaris Riesenberg, Ronen Toledano, Francisc Schlaeffer,

Alexander Smolyakov, Lisa Saidel-Odes, Oded Wechsberg, Jacob N. Ablin, Victor Novack, and Dan Buskila. "Prevalence and Characteristics of Fibromyalgia among HIV-Positive Patients in Southern Israel." *Clinical and Experimental Rheumatology* 34, no. 2 (March–April 2016): S34–9.

Ford, Brett Q., Phoebe Lam, Oliver P. John, and Iris B. Mauss. "The Psychological Health Benefits of Accepting Negative Emotions and Thoughts: Laboratory, Diary, and Longitudinal Evidence." *Journal of Personality and Social Psychology* 115, no. 6 (July 2018): 1075–92. doi:10.1037/pspp0000157.

Genkinger, Jeanine M, and Anita Koushik. "Meat Consumption and Cancer Risk." *PLoS Medicine* 4, no. 12 (December 2007): e345. doi:10.1371/journal.pmed.0040345.

Glombiewski, Julia Anna, Kathrin Bernardy, and Winfried Häuser. "Efficacy of EMG- and EEG-Biofeedback in Fibromyalgia Syndrome: A Meta-Analysis and a Systematic Review of Randomized Controlled Trials." *Evidence-Based Complementary and Alternative Medicine* (September 2013). doi:10.1155/2013/962741.

Goebel, A., S. Buhner, R. Schedel, H. Lochs, and G. Sprotte. "Altered Intestinal Permeability in Patients with Primary Fibromyalgia and in Patients with Complex Regional Pain Syndrome." *Rheumatology* 47, no. 8 (August 2008): 1223–7. doi:10.1093/rheumatology/ken140.

Goldenberg, D. L., L. A. Bradley, L. M. Arnold, and J. M. Glass. "Understanding Fibromyalgia and Its Related Disorders." Primary Care Companion to the Journal of Clinical Psychiatry 10, no. 2 (January 2008): 133–44. doi:10.4088/pcc.v10n0208.

Gordon, William Van, Edo Shonin, Thomas J. Dunn, Javier Garcia-Campayo, and Mark D. Griffiths. "Meditation Awareness Training for the Treatment of Fibromyalgia Syndrome: A Randomized Controlled Trial." *British Journal of Health Psychology* 22, no. 1 (February 2017): 186–206. doi:10.1111/bjhp.12224.

Gowans, Susan E. and Amy deHueck. "Tips for Starting a Program for Your Patients—Exercise for Fibromyalgia: Benefits and Practical Advice." *The Journal of Musculoskeletal Medicine* 23, no. 9 (September 2006): 614.

Gui, Maísa Soares, Marcele Jardim Pimentel, and Célia Marisa Rizzatti-Barbosa. "Temporomandibular Disorders in Fibromyalgia Syndrome: A Short-Communication." *Revista Brasileira de Reumatologia* 55, no. 2 (March-April 2015): 189-94. doi: 10.1016/j.rbr.2014.07.004.

Hannibal, Kara E. and Mark D. Bishop. "Chronic Stress, Cortisol Dysfunction, and Pain: A Psychoneuroendocrine Rationale for Stress Management in Pain Rehabilitation." *Physical Therapy* 94, no. 12 (December 2014): 1816–25. doi:10.2522/ptj.20130597.

Hart, Archibald D. *Adrenaline and Stress.* Nashville, TN: Thomas Nelson, 1995.

Harvard Health Publications. "Blue Light Has a Dark Side." Last modified August 13, 2018. Health.Harvard.edu/staying-healthy/blue-light-has-a-dark-side.

Harvard Health Publications. "Try a FODMAPs Diet to Manage Irritable Bowel Syndrome." Last modified September 17, 2019. Health.Harvard.edu/diet-and-weight-loss/a-new-diet-to-manage-irritable-bowel-syndrome.

Häuser, Winfried, Brian Walitt, Mary-Ann Fitzcharles, and Claudia Sommer. "Review of Pharmacological Therapies in Fibromyalgia Syndrome." *Arthritis Research & Therapy* 16, no. 1 (January 2014): 201. doi:10.1186/ar4441.

Honda, Yuichiro, Junya Sakamoto, Yohei Hamaue, Hideki Kataoka, Yasutaka Kondo, Ryo Sasabe, Kyo Goto, Takuya Fukushima, Satoshi Oga, Ryo Sasaki, Natsumi Tanaka, Jiro Nakano, and Minoru Okita. "Effects of Physical-Agent Pain Relief Modalities for Fibromyalgia Patients: A Systematic Review and Meta-Analysis of Randomized Controlled Trials." *Pain Research and Management* 2018 (October 2018): 1–9. doi:10.1155/2018/2930632.

Kaluza, Joanna, Agneta Åkesson, and Alicja Wolk. "Processed

and Unprocessed Red Meat Consumption and Risk of Heart Failure." *Circulation: Heart Failure* 7, no. 4 (July 2014): 552–7. doi:10.1161 /circheartfailure.113.000921.

Kenny, Brian J. and Bruno Bordoni. "Neuroanatomy, Cranial Nerve 10 (Vagus Nerve)." *Stat*Pearls. Last modified January 25, 2020. NCBI.NLM.NIH.gov/books /NBK537171.

Köseoğlu, Handan İnönü, Ahmet İnanır, Asiye Kanbay, Sevil Okan, Osman Demir, Osman Çeçen, and Sema İnanır. "Is There a Link between Obstructive Sleep Apnea Syndrome and Fibromyalgia Syndrome?" *Turkish Thoracic Journal* 18, no. 2 (April 2017): 40–6. doi:10.5152/ TurkThoracJ.2017.16036.

Kozanoglu, Erkan, Abdullah Canataroglu, Bahri Abayli, Salih Colakoglu, and Kamil Goncu. "Fibromyalgia Syndrome in Patients with Hepatitis C Infection." *Rheumatology International* 23, no. 5 (September 2003): 248–51. doi:10.1007 /s00296-003-0290-7.

Kunnumakkara, Ajaikumar B., Bethsebie L. Sailo, Kishore Banik, Choudhary Harsha, Sahdeo Prasad, Subash Chandra Gupta, Alok Chandra Bharti, and Bharat B. Aggarwal. "Chronic Diseases, Inflammation, and Spices: How Are They Linked?" *Journal of Translational Medicine* 16, no. 1 (January 2018): 14. doi:10.1186 /s12967-018-1381-2.

Kunz, Barbara and Kevin. "Reflexology Techniques." *Complete Reflexology for Life.* London: DK Publishing, 2009.

Kwiatek, Richard. "Treatment of Fibromyalgia." *Australian Prescriber* 40, no. 5 (October 2017): 179–83. doi:10.18773 /austprescr.2017.056.

Kwon, Chan-Young and Boram Lee. "Acupuncture or Acupressure on Yintang (EX-HN 3) for Anxiety: A Preliminary Review." *Medical Acupuncture* 30, no. 2 (April 2018): 73–9. doi: 10.1089 /acu.2017.1268.

Lakhan, Shaheen E., Heather Sheafer, and Deborah Tepper. "The Effectiveness of Aromatherapy in Reducing Pain: A Systematic Review and

Meta-Analysis." *Pain Research and Treatment* 2016, no. 7 (January 2016): 1–13. doi:10.1155/2016/8158693.

Lankarani, Kamran B. "Diet and the Gut." *Middle East Journal of Digestive Diseases* 8, no. 3 (July 2016): 161–5. doi:10.15171/mejdd.2016.28.

Li, Yan-hui, et al. "Massage Therapy for Fibromyalgia: A Systematic Review and Meta-Analysis of Randomized Controlled Trials." *PLoS One* 9, no. 2 (February 2014): e89304. doi:10.1371/journal.pone.0089304.

Linnemann, Alexandra, Mattes B. Kappert, Susanne Fischer, Johanna M. Doerr, Jana Strahler, and Urs M. Nater. "The Effects of Music Listening on Pain and Stress in the Daily Life of Patients with Fibromyalgia Syndrome." *Frontiers in Human Neuroscience* 9 (July 2015): 434. doi:10.3389/fnhum.2015.00434.

Lipski, Elizabeth. "Coming Back into Balance." In *Digestive Wellness: Strengthen the Immune System and Prevent Disease through Healthy Digestion*, 4th ed. New York: McGraw-Hill, 2011.

Meeus, Mira, Jo Nijs, Linda Hermans, Dorien Goubert, and Patrick Calders. "The Role of Mitochondrial Dysfunctions Due to Oxidative and Nitrosative Stress in the Chronic Pain or Chronic Fatigue Syndromes and Fibromyalgia Patients: Peripheral and Central Mechanisms as Therapeutic Targets?" *Expert Opinion on Therapeutic Targets* 17, no. 9 (September 2013): 1081–9. doi:10.1517/14728222.2013.818657.

Miranda, Renata Costa De, Eduardo S. Paiva, Silvia Maria Suter Correia Cadena, Anna Paula Brandt, and Regina Maria Vilela. "Polyphenol-Rich Foods Alleviate Pain and Ameliorate Quality of Life in Fibromyalgic Women." *International Journal for Vitamin and Nutrition Research* 87, no. 1–2 (March 2017): 66–74. doi:10.1024/0300-9831/a000253.

Morhenn, Vera, Laura E. Beavin and Paul Zak. "Massage Increases Oxytocin and Reduces Adrenocorticotropin Hormone in Humans." *Alternative Therapies in Health and Medicine* 18, no. 6 (November-December 2012): 11–18.

Nascimento, Simone De Souza, Josimari Melo Desantana, Fernando Kenji Nampo, Êurica Adélia Nogueira Ribeiro, Daniel Lira da Silva, João Xavier Araújo-Júnior, Jackson Roberto Guedes da Silva Almeida, Leonardo Rigoldi Bonjardim, Adriano Antunes de Souza Araújo, and Lucindo José Quintans-Júnior. "Efficacy and Safety of Medicinal Plants or Related Natural Products for Fibromyalgia: A Systematic Review." *Evidence-Based Complementary and Alternative Medicine* 2013 (June 2013): 1–10. doi:10.1155/2013/149468.

National Institutes of Health. "Omega-3 Fatty Acids." Accessed April 24, 2020. ODS.OD.NIH .gov/factsheets/Omega3Fatty Acids-Consumer.

National Institute of Neurological Disorders and Stroke. "Brain Basics: Understanding Sleep." Accessed April 24, 2020. NINDS. NIH.gov/Disorders/Patient -Caregiver-Education /Understanding-Sleep.

Neeck, G. and W. Riedel. "Thyroid Function in Patients with Fibromyalgia Syndrome." *The Journal of Rheumatology* 19, no. 7 (July 1992): 1120–2.

Olendzki, Barbara, and Jennifer Chaiken. "Using Black Pepper to Enhance the Anti-Inflammatory Effects of Turmeric." *UMass Medical School Center for Applied Nutrition* (blog). June 28, 2019. UMassMed.edu/nutrition /blog/blog-posts/2019/6/using -blackpepper-to-enhance -the-anti-inflammatoryeffects -of-turmeric.

Reshkova, V., Ivan G. Milanov, and Desislava Kalinova. "Evaluation of Antiviral Antibodies against Epstein-Barr Virus and Neurotransmitters in Patients with Fibromyalgia." *Journal of Neurology and Neuroscience* 6, no. 3 (November 14, 2015). doi: 10.21767/2171-6625.100035.

Rhee, H. J. van der, Esther de Vries, and Jan Willem W. Coebergh. "Regular Sun Exposure Benefits Health." *Medical Hypotheses* 97, 19 (October 2016): 34–7. doi:10.1016/j.mehy.2016.10.011.

Ricciotti, Hope and Hye-Chun Hur. "Do Fish Oil Supplements Reduce Inflammation?" *Harvard*

Women's Health Watch. Published September 2016. Health. Harvard.edu/staying -healthy/do-fish-oil-supplements -reduce-inflammation.

Riva, Roberto, Paul Jarle Mork, Rolf Harald Westgaard, Magne Rø, and Ulf Lundberg. "Fibromyalgia Syndrome Is Associated with Hypocortisolism." *International Journal of Behavioral Medicine* 17, no. 3 (May 2010): 223–33. doi:10.1007/s12529-010-9097-6.

Sañudo, Borja, Delfín Galiano, Luis Carrasco, Moisés de Hoyo, and Joseph G. McVeigh. "Effects of a Prolonged Exercise Program on Key Health Outcomes in Women with Fibromyalgia: A Randomized Controlled Trial." *Journal of Rehabilitation Medicine* 43, no. 6 (May 2011): 521–6. doi:10.2340/16501977-0814.

Schertzinger, Meredith, Kate Wesson-Sides, Luke Parkitny, and Jarred Younger. "Daily Fluctuations of Progesterone and Testosterone Are Associated with Fibromyalgia Pain Severity." *The Journal of Pain* 19, no. 4 (April 2018): 410–7. doi:10.1016/j. jpain.2017.11.013.

Silva, Ana Rita, Alexandra Bernardo, João Costa, Alexandra Cardoso, Paula Santos, Maria Fernanda de Mesquita, José Vaz Patto, Pedro Moreira, Maria Leonor Silva, and Patrícia Padrão. "Dietary Interventions in Fibromyalgia: a Systematic Review." *Annals of Medicine* 51, suppl. 1 (February 2019): 2–14. doi:10.1080 /07853890.2018.1564360.

Singh, Rabindarjeet. "The Importance of Exercise as a Therapeutic Agent." *The Malaysian Journal of Medical Sciences* 9, no. 2 (July 2002): 7–16. NCBI.NLM .NIH.gov/pmc/articles /PMC3406202.

Smyth, Joshua M., Jillian A. Johnson, Brandon J. Auer, Erik Lehman, Giampaolo Talamo, and Christopher N. Sciamanna. "Online Positive Affect Journaling in the Improvement of Mental Distress and Well-Being in General Medical Patients with Elevated Anxiety Symptoms: A Preliminary Randomized Controlled Trial." *JMIR Mental Health* 5, no. 4 (December 2018): e11290. doi:10.2196/11290.

Sosa-Reina, M. Dolores, Susana Nunez-Nagy, Tomás

Gallego-Izquierdo, Daniel Pecos-Martín, Jorge Monserrat, and Melchor Álvarez-Mon. "Effectiveness of Therapeutic Exercise in Fibromyalgia Syndrome: A Systematic Review and Meta-Analysis of Randomized Clinical Trials." *BioMed Research International* 2017 (September 2017). doi: 10.1155/2017/2356346.

Terry, Rohini, Rachel Perry, and Edzard Ernst. "An Overview of Systematic Reviews of Complementary and Alternative Medicine for Fibromyalgia." *Clinical Rheumatology* 31, no. 1 (January 2012): 55–66. doi:10.1007/s10067-011-1783-5.

Thiel, Robert J. *Naturopathy for the 21st Century: Combining Old and New*. Warsaw, IN: W Whitman Publications, 2001.

Trudeau, Michelle. "Human Connections Start with a Friendly Touch." NPR. September 20, 2010. NPR.org/templates/story /story.php?storyId=128795325.

United States Geological Survey. "The Water in You: Water and the Human Body." Accessed April 24, 2020. USGS.gov/special-topic /water-scienceschool/science /wateryou-water-and-human body?qt-science_center _objects=0#qt-science _center_objects.

Viola-Saltzman, Mari, Nathaniel F. Watson, Andy Bogart, Jack Goldberg, and Dedra Buchwald. "High Prevalence of Restless Legs Syndrome among Patients with Fibromyalgia: A Controlled Cross-Sectional Study." *Journal of Clinical Sleep Medicine* 6, no. 5 (October 2010): 423–7. NCBI .NLM.NIH.gov/pmc/articles /PMC2952743.

Walitt, Brian, Richard L. Nahin, Robert S. Katz, Martin J. Bergman, and Frederick Wolfe. "The Prevalence and Characteristics of Fibromyalgia in the 2012 National Health Interview Survey." *PLoS One* 10, no. 9 (September 2015): e0138024. doi:10.1371/journal. pone.0138024.

White, Kevin P., Simon Carette, Manfred Harth, and Robert W. Teasell. "Trauma and Fibromyalgia: Is There an Association and What Does It Mean?" *Seminars in Arthritis and Rheumatism*

29, no. 4 (February 2000): 200–16. doi:10.1016/s0049-0172(00)80009-8.

Wise, Norman R. "Proactive Perspective." *Succeeding at Life: Living a Sane, Stable, and Spiritual Life.* Redeemer Publishing, 2010.

Zügel, Martina, Constantinos N. Maganaris, Jan Wilke, Karin Jurkat-Rott, Werner Klingler, Scott C. Wearing, Thomas Findley, Mary F. Barbe, Jürgen Michael Steinacker, Andry Vleeming, Wilhelm Bloch, Robert Schleip, and Paul William Hodges. "Fascial Tissue Research in Sports Medicine: from Molecules to Tissue Adaptation, Injury and Diagnostics: Consensus Statement." *British Journal of Sports Medicine* 52, no. 23 (August 2018): 1497. doi:10.1136/bjsports-2018-099308.

Zwickey, Heather, Angela Horgan, Doug Hanes, Heather Schiffke, Annie Moore, Helané Wahbeh, Julia Jordan, Lila Ojeda, Martha McMurry, Patricia Elmer, and Jonathan Q. Purnell. "Effect of the Anti-Inflammatory Diet in People with Diabetes and Pre-Diabetes: A Randomized Controlled Feeding Study." *Journal of Restorative Medicine* 8, no.1 (June 2019): e20190107. doi:10.14200/jrm.2019.0107.

INDEX

ACKNOWLEDGMENTS

I thank God for providing me with this opportunity to give others hope and tools to improve their current health.

To the most vital people to my healing journey: Dr. Jennifer Hastings, Phyllis Wright, Dr. Norman Wise, and others. Thank you for allowing God to use you in His process of molding a healthier and more sane, stable, and spiritual version of myself. It was necessary for me to go through everything I went through to become the woman I am today and help others who may be going through the same. I have learned a great deal from you all and hope to continue passing that knowledge along.

To my family, and most specifically my mother, Aurea, thank you. You are the ones who put up with me and stepped in to help out with my other responsibilities so that I could write this book quickly. Thank you for being my unconditional supporters and motivators. Mami, thank you for being a nanny, a personal assistant, a chef, and all the other hats you wear to come to my rescue.

Thank you to Clara Song Lee, Andrea Leptinsky, Katherine Green, and the rest of the team at Rockridge Press for giving me this wonderful opportunity to write a book that I hope and pray will be a blessing to many. Thank you as well for your guidance and support throughout the process. The behind-the-scenes team oftentimes works the hardest and gets the least recognition. This journey has been exciting and has taught me a great deal. Thank you for all your hard work.

ABOUT THE AUTHOR

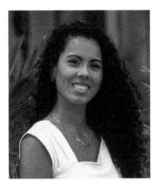 **Dr. Amarilis Méndez** is a traditional naturopath and owner of Counter Cultural Health. She has a bachelor's degree in biology, a master's degree in public health, and she's a licensed naturopath. She is also certified in integrative and functional medicine. After being diagnosed with several chronic conditions, including fibromyalgia, she decided not to continue her pursuit of an allopathic medical degree; instead, she studied the natural healing arts. Once her symptoms were resolved, she began her journey to educate others about their bodies' natural healing abilities and what they can do to enhance it.

Now she serves out of her practice, offering face-to-face and remote holistic consultations. In her work, she helps her clients incorporate clinical nutrition, orthomolecular nutrition, herbal medicine, functional medicine, aromatherapy, applied kinesiology, lifestyle coaching, and counseling.

For more information about her philosophy and the different services she provides, you can visit CCHealing.com.